*Caring for Elderly People
in the Community*

Caring for Elderly People in the Community

Second edition

E. Idris Williams
Professor of General Practice,
The University of Nottingham.

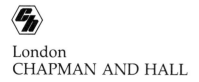

London
CHAPMAN AND HALL

First published in 1979 by Croom Helm Ltd

Second edition 1989 by Chapman and Hall Ltd
11 New Fetter Lane, London EC4P 4EE

© 1979, 1989 E. Idris Williams

Typeset in 10 on 12 pt Palatino by
Best-set Typesetter Limited, Hong Kong
Printed in Great Britain by
T.J. Press (Padstow) Ltd,
Padstow, Cornwall

ISBN 0 412 32650 7

British Library Cataloguing in Publication Data

Williams, Idris
  Caring for elderly people in the community.
  – 2nd ed.
  1. Great Britain. Old persons. Care
  I. Title   II. Williams, Idris. The care of the
  elderly in the community.
  362.6'0941

ISBN 0-412-32650-7

Contents

Preface

The first edition of this book was based on my experiences of twenty years as a family doctor. In part, it traced my developing understanding of the natural history of ageing in the community and the real needs of old people living at home. Out of this grew a strategy of preventive medicine which, at that time, essentially meant screening entire practice populations of over-75-year olds. The emphasis has now changed and widened. Throughout the world there is an increasing recognition of the special needs of old people and to meet these, many countries are developing programmes with a specific focus on care in the community. This has meant that in the past decade there have been many developments in community and family care and these are incorporated into this new edition. The basic objectives of such care remain, however, very much as they were; the main one being to keep old people self-supportive and independent. The need to preserve functional ability has if anything become more important. Maintaining quality of life has always been a prime objective of the professional services and to achieve this it has been necessary to encourage positive attitudes towards old age and reject a nihilistic approach. The need to take account of the wishes of elderly people themselves has also always been important. These basic principles of caring for the elders remain valid and contribute to the underlying philosophy of this book.

Despite some attempts at institutional care for sick and destitute old people, some dating back to the Middle Ages, most of the care provided for elderly persons has always taken place in the home. The responsibility for this care has rested with the family and medical attention has usually been provided by the general practitioner or family physician together with domiciliary nurses. In the UK this pattern of medical care was perpetuated by the National Health Service when health visiting, district nursing and general-practitioner care were made freely available to all, including old people in their homes. By the 1950s when departments of geriatric medicine were being established in hospitals, it also became clear that nursing of many chronically ill old persons was taking place within the community itself. An early pioneer, J.H. Sheldon, when calling for changes in the care of old people in hospital, also drew attention to the plight of old people in their own homes (Sheldon, 1971).

He thought it might be necessary to provide a special community geriatric medical service and pointed to the severe strain imposed on younger generations in caring for elderly people. He did not mention the general practitioner and other members of the community-care team as possible providers of care and it is significant that his comments were made at a time when community services were at a low point in the UK – shortly after the introduction of the National Health Service. However, since then the importance of community care complementary to, and in partnership with, hospital care has been appreciated and developed. This book does not advocate a specific geriatric service operating in the community, but a primary-care service, which regards old people as normal members of the community and not medically segregated to be treated differently. It also recognizes that particularly for the over-75-year olds, there are opportunities for prevention, maintenance and rehabilitation, which can realistically improve the quality of life.

Despite the development of professional care, the family continues to provide most of the care needed in the community. This means increasingly heavy demands on husbands, wives, brothers, sisters, children and even more distant relatives and friends. Many studies have shown the intensity of the strain on carers and it is clear that they too demand special consideration and support within the community. Their needs will be discussed at various points throughout this book.

The purpose of this book is therefore to describe domiciliary care for elderly people in its widest sense. It is not a textbook of geriatric medicine, but rather a complementary work that concerns itself with what happens outside the domain of secondary care. Chapters 2–5 set the scene with an up-to-date description of the demographic, social, economic and health status of elderly people in the community. This provides information about the background to life in old age and a database for planning family-care initiatives. Chapters 6 and 7 describe the dynamics of health in association with ageing and the very important social interactions involved. Chapters 8 and 9 outline health- and social-care provisions in the community. This includes a careful definition of objectives. New initiatives are examined and special attention is given to the importance of the family as carers. Chapters 10–13 review developments in preventive care and the options available are critically examined. Assessment of old persons has a rapidly growing international and interdisciplinary importance. A recent working party set up by the Kellogg Foundation and the World Health Organization has clarified many of the issues that were outstanding. The guidelines laid down by this working party are closely followed in Chapter 14. In Chapter 15 the hospital–community interface is described and new guidelines for discharging patients from hospital and receiving them back into the community are presented. This is an important new area where initiatives are urgently needed. The management of patients with long-term medical problems is linked to this important area.

Chapters 16–18 consider the old person in family practice and describe the medical and nursing responses. The principles will be of relevance to primary care in both developed and developing countries. Chapter 19 describes some of the common difficulties in the community. Using a problem-solving approach it gives a practical multidisciplinary description of management of important conditions outside hospital. Over the past few years the ethical dilemmas confronting community workers involved with old people have also been recognized and these are described in Chapter 20. The important contribution of community care for the dying patient is reviewed in Chapter 21. Finally, in the conclusion, a discussion takes place on the importance of education for all those involved in caring for elderly people. This is now recognized by the inclusion in most medical schools of experience at undergraduate level in health care of elderly people. Trainee general practitioners and family doctors are also expected to gain experience in caring for old people. In the UK the newly instituted Diploma in Geriatric Medicine of the Royal College of Physicians is an important development to stimulate educational developments. This book takes into account these educational needs.

Although this work is intended primarily for members of the community-care team, it is also designed for those people caring for an old person at home. Some of the chapters are, of necessity, technical and will have more relevance for the professional reader. My experience is, however, that carers and patients themselves do want to know more about the illness and I hope that the more clinical chapters will be useful to them.

There are therefore several different types of reader: the professional carers (doctors, nurses, social workers, physiotherapists, occupational therapists, speech therapists and indeed all members of the team together with the students of these professions), family members, members of voluntary organizations and very importantly, the reception staff at surgeries and health centres. The book may be of interest to teachers who are concerned with educating children about the services available in the community. It is important that young people gain an insight into what old age is really like. Many grandchildren do become the prime carers of old people. I realize that in aiming at so wide a group of readers I may not satisfy any one of them. The danger is obvious, but as so many people are involved in looking after the aged the risk is probably worth taking.

The book will also be relevant in countries other than the UK. Experience has shown that in every society the care of old persons in their homes raises the same issues and although methods of delivering care may vary from place to place, the basic natural history and the problems presented are very similar in most countries. The recent developments in the United States of America, where family medicine is taking a fuller role in looking after old persons, are of course very relevant.

The book inevitably reflects my own philosophy towards old people and their care. I have a positive and practical approach: taking action where life can be improved or saved, but not interfering unnecessarily. I try to look at the situation through the old person's eyes. I have researched many of these areas myself and am very aware of situations that need further clarification. I do not see the care of elderly people as separate from the mainstream of medical care, particularly so in the community. I believe that there should be a close co-operation between those looking after old people in hospital and in the community. They are essentially part of the same process and should link closely together in the provision of services.

The recent government White Paper *Working for Patients* is likely to form the basis of legislation which will affect both hospital and general practitioner services. Many of the proposals concern the provision of care for old people. Comments about these changes and their possible impact are made at appropriate points in the book. However the basic principles of care will remain the same.

REFERENCE

Sheldon J.H. (1971) A history of British geriatrics. *Modern Geriatrics*, **1**, (7), 330–5.

Foreword

Professor Idris Williams must be congratulated on producing a book which is so relevant to the many people caring for the old in their own homes and at the same time is so encyclopaedic in its content. *Caring for Elderly People in the Community* is easy to read, extremely well documented with tables and graphs and discusses almost every topic that those looking after old people will want to know about – be they doctors, nurses, informal carers or, indeed, elderly people themselves. To produce a work of such wide appeal which the professionals will find stimulating and scholarly, is no mean feat and I believe Professor Williams has been extremely successful in his task.

The work spans the field from demography to ethics via the biological, clinical and organizational aspects of old age. The chapters are all authoritative and those which reflect the author's particular research interests (such as assessment, screening and prevention) are outstanding.

Idris Williams is one of the small number of family practitioners who has special interest in, and knowledge of, old age. He has blazed a trail in this field and it is now clear that more and more of his colleagues are following in his footsteps. This must be, since the general practitioner should always be the cornerstone of care for the ever increasing number of old people in our nation. This book is commended as a work which will encourage this development, and supply a factual basis for its growth.

J.C. Brocklehurst, CBE, MD, FRCP
Professor of Geriatric Medicine
University of Manchester

Acknowledgements

I would like to thank John Bendall, Peter Hope, Jane Iliffe, Edith Elliot, Alan Murphy, Lynne Cater, Nick Galloway, Kevin Gibbin, John Temple and Richard Beaver for reading parts of the manuscript and making very helpful comments. I used some material from projects written by medical students John Somauroo and Gavin Darbyshire in Chapter 5 and would like to acknowledge their help in giving me permission to do this. Charles Freer and Chris Smith gave me invaluable help in reading and correcting the whole manuscript. Their comments and criticisms were greatly appreciated and I am very much in their debt. I am grateful to Elizabeth R. Perkins for permission to quote from her literature review of preventive care for the elderly. I am grateful also to Lindsay Groom for cataloguing the references and Ann Zamorski for drafting the figures. Finally, I must thank Alison Slater and Judy Rose for the painstaking work they have done in turning my illegible manuscript into a beautifully typed finished work.

1 *International scene*

Although most elders in developed countries are in reasonably good health and enjoy an independent life, the very fact that in most of these countries there is a rapidly growing elderly population can bring with it challenges. The increase in the number of patients with chronic illness and the reservoir of unreported need experienced in all societies means that elderly people fairly universally need special arrangements for health and social care. The organizational responses to these special needs, however, differ from country to country (Nusberg, *et al.* 1984).

FINANCIAL SYSTEMS

With the exception of the USA most countries provide health care for their older people through the same system that serves all age groups. The United Kingdom National Health Service is a good example of this. The advantage of this system is that it integrates health care of elderly people with that provided for other age groups and lessens the risks of segregating such care and perhaps providing a second-class service. National services, funded mainly through general revenues, are a standard way of delivering health care in socialist countries such as the USSR and the German Democratic Republic, and also exist in the UK and Italy. National insurance programmes, financed largely through employer/employee contributions, exist in most of the market economies, such as France, the Federal German Republic and Sweden. Many countries, however, have a combination of health-care financing services, although one tends to dominate. In the USA for instance, although medical care is mainly funded through private insurance, because of difficulties in providing such care for elderly people in that system, Medicare, a state-funded system, was introduced. Although national health services and insurance programmes do seem to provide more adequate coverage than do private systems, the services provided for elderly people in all countries have their own inadequacies. These include shortage of personnel and shortfalls in the levels of various aspects of the service provided. Although there are often special arrangements for elderly persons, for example, free prescriptions in the UK, there are pressures to keep these to a minimum. In the UK, however, the increased workload associated with caring for older people is recognized by additional fees being paid to the general practitioner for patients over 65 years old, with a further increase for those over 75 years of age. The difficulty associated with charging a fee to an old person at the time of need is that it accentuates the well-known tendency of failure to report that need. The end result is delay, thus allowing problems to become worse and so producing even greater pressure on the system.

Long-term care is another area where systems in different countries vary. Medicare coverage for either nursing or community care is very limited in the USA. In France, nursing-home residents are expected to contribute towards their room and board. In the UK there is now emerging a mixed system with both local authority and privately owned homes. The private system is, however, also state-supported through the Social Security system.

The proportion of the gross national product (GNP) spent on health care in industrialized societes varies considerably; the UK for instance spends proportionately about half as much as the USA. Despite the large differences in relative expenditure, there does not seem to be any difference between the two systems in terms of health-status indicators in the elderly population.

COMMUNITY HEALTH SERVICES

General practitioners or family doctors are often the first point of contact with the health services for older people. However, when planning services for elderly people, these doctors have to a certain extent been bypassed, often because of lack of training and general disinterest amongst the doctors themselves. But in most countries the important role of the family physician has now been recognized and special training is being provided. Home visiting to old people by family doctors has almost disappeared in many countries, although in the UK and the USSR these visits are still continuing. In Britain two-thirds of consultations with patients over 75 years old are at home. Home nursing exists in all developed countries although with differing degrees of adequacy. In some countries, for example, Czechoslovakia, there are 'geriatric nurses' who are responsible for home nursing of old people. In the USA this provision is not fully developed. It is likely that most countries will have to develop a systematic care programme for old people in the community, if only for the reason that secondary care in hospital will prove to be far too expensive an alternative. The place of preventive health measures as part of community care is still uncertain, but because of escalating costs, interest in such measures is increasing everywhere. General health-promotion initiatives are, for instance, being introduced in Scandinavia, the USSR, the Federal Republic of Germany and the Netherlands. These usually involve special health education about exercise, fitness, diet and so on. Secondary prevention has also attracted interest with preparation for retirement and regular health checks are also proving popular. Internationally, however, there is still uncertainty about routine assessment programmes.

REFERENCE

Nusberg, C. Gibson, M.J. and Peace, S. (1984) *Innovative Aging Programs Abroad. Implications for the United States*, Greenwood Press, Connecticut and London.

2 *Demographic trends*

The demographic pattern of old age is continually changing. Census returns over the last century show that the elderly populations of over 65 and of over 75 have increased dramatically both in actual numbers and in proportion to the total population (see Table 2.1). This is essentially due to both mortality and fertility factors. Declining infant- and child-mortality rates have produced a larger proportion of cohorts now surviving to adulthood and going on to become elderly. So although the life expectancy in 1987 at the age of 60 was not radically different from that in 1900, the proportion of any cohort reaching 60 is now much higher, so the life-expectancy figure at birth is much improved. There was a major decline in marital fertility in England and Wales in the period between the 1870s and the 1930s. Thus, with declining birth input into the demographic system the relative size of the elderly group was increased. This explains the increase in both numbers and proportion of elderly people in the population today.

The present age structure of the population in Great Britain at the last census which was in 1981 is shown in Table 2.2. The drop in numbers after the age of 80 is noteworthy: to reach this age and beyond is still an achievement. The actual numbers of old people over 80 years old and their relative proportion to the rest of the population is still quite low despite the enormous relative increase over the past few decades. A model of the demographic age and sex distribution for 1981 is shown in Fig. 2.1. The life expectancy at birth in this year was for men 69.73 years, and for women 75.68 years. The contrast in the shape of the model of life expectation between 1981, 1951, 1921, 1901 and 1851 is dramatic.

The number of people reaching 100 years of age also increased from 200 in 1952 to 1750 in 1982. The reasons for this are complex but include a higher absolute number of births in 1882 than 1852 (despite a falling birth rate) coupled with mortality and migration characteristics that were different for the two cohort groups (Smith and Ebrahim, 1984).

The structure of the elderly population by age, sex and marital status is shown in Table 2.3. In all age bands women outnumber men, and increasingly so as age advances. The numbers of divorced elderly people are still very small although this could increase enormously over the next two or three decades. Currently, the divorced make up only 1% of the

Table 2.1 Population trends over the last century (England and Wales)

Age	1851		1901		1931		1971		1981	
	n (mill)	%	n (mill)	%	n (mill)	%	n (mill)	%	n (mill)	%
65+	0.65	3.60	1.50	4.60	3.00	7.50	6.35	12.96	7.27	14.84
75+	0.15	0.83	0.50	1.53	0.90	2.25	2.35	4.80	2.79	5.69
Total population	18	100	32.6	100	40	100	49	100	49	100

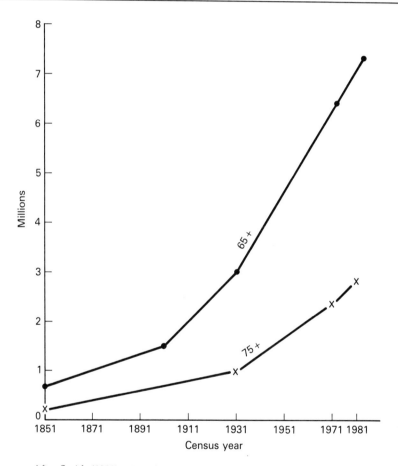

Source: After Smith (1988) using data from censuses for 1851–1981

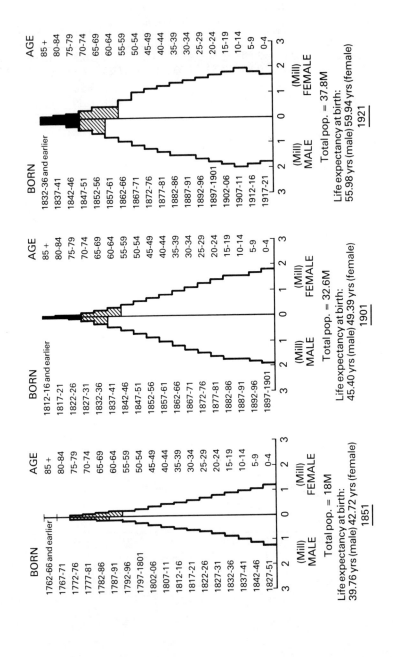

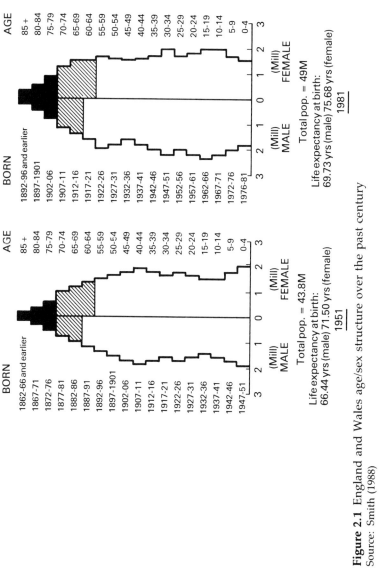

Figure 2.1 England and Wales age/sex structure over the past century
Source: Smith (1988)

Table 2.2 Present population age/sex structure. Great Britain 1981 census

Total population:	53 556 911	(100%)
Total age 65+:	7 985 102	(15%)
Total age 75+:	3 052 795	(6%)
Total age 85+:	552 387	(1%)
Age/sex distribution		
Age	Male	Female
65–69 years	1 205 583	1 461 459
70–79 years	1 549 033	2 317 085
80–89 years	368 642	924 190
90+ years	31 990	127 120

Source: OPCS (1983a)

elderly population, compared with the general level of marriages ending in divorce of 33%.

In all major regions of the world women outnumber men in old age but the number of men per thousand women varies significantly (see Table 2.4). In South Asia the number of men per thousand women is high, perhaps due to the poorer status of women or higher maternal mortality. The lower proportion of males in Europe is the result of several factors: the lower life expectancy of men, male casualties in two world wars and emigration of young males in the early part of the century. The especially low proportion in the USSR is likely to be the result of large World War II casualties and earlier political purges.

There are of course regional and local variations. It seems to be a characteristic of many cities, especially in developed countries, that there is a concentration of elderly people in the inner cities. For instance, in Nottingham, England, the proportion of elderly people in the inner-city area is nearly 20% in some areas. There is a movement of younger people out to the suburbs. Economic forces prevent elderly people from moving and social restraints reinforce this.

It is very difficult to place elderly persons in a social class and the previous employment of the head of household does not necessarily equate with living standards in old age. The figures quoted in the 1981 census are shown in Table 2.5. There are differences in the way in which the 1971 and 1981 censuses dealt with social class in elderly people. However, if allowance is made for this there is some evidence that Social Classes I, II and III (non-manual) are increasing their size proportionately and groups IV and V (manual) are declining.

Similar trends in the population of over 65s are seen in most developed countries. The USA for instance shows a peaking in overall numbers and also a change in balance. East Germany now has over 16% of persons over 65 and in this respect is the most elderly nation in the world,

Table 2.3 Structure of elderly population (65+ years) by age, sex and marital status. Great Britain 1978

	Males		Females	
	(millions)	*(%)*	*(millions)*	*(%)*
Married	2.3	74.2	1.7	34.7
Single	0.3	9.7	0.5	10.2
Widowed/divorced	0.5	16.1	2.7	55.1
Total	3.1	100	4.9	100

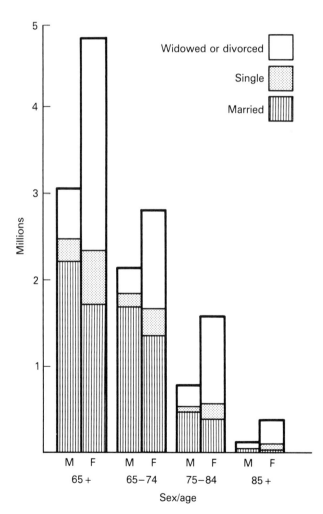

Source: DHSS (1983)

Table 2.4 Males per 1000 females by age
group and major world regions, 1975

Region	Age (years)	
	(75–79)	(80+)
Africa	783	748
Latin America	802	705
North America	637	558
East Asia	790	685
South Asia	959	863
Europe	595	486
Oceania	686	525
USSR	410	382

Source: Grundy (1983)

Table 2.5 Change in social-class structure in Great Britain – numbers of
households. Ten per cent sample.

Social class	1971		1981	
I	74 563	(5.35%)	74 944	(5.93%)
II	270 414	(19.39%)	321 796	(25.46%)
III (non-manual)	159 705	(11.45%)	175 679	(13.90%)
III (manual)	533 936	(38.28%)	414 215	(32.77%)
IV	248 315	(17.80%)	208 493	(16.50%)
V	107 861	(7.73%)	68 835	(5.45%)
Total	1 394 794	(100%)	1 263 962	(100%)

Source: OPCS (1975; 1983b)

closely followed by Sweden and West Germany. The German Democratic
Republic has this high proportion of elderly people primarily as a result of
very low fertility amongst married couples today. Emigration of elderly
people to the Federal Republic of Germany is not discouraged by the East
German Government. The total world trends are seen in Fig. 2.2.

At the local level a practice population of 2200 patients could expect to
have 328 over-65-year-old patients of which 131 would be male and 197
would be female. Within this group there would be 125 over-75-year olds
(41 male and 84 female) and 23 over-85-year olds (5 male and 18 female).
There are, however, variations depending upon locality and region.

The future trends in the elderly population numbers and proportions
are interesting and represent a change in outlook. It appears likely that a
peaking of numbers of the over 65s in England and Wales will soon
occur and may even be happening now. Between now and the year 2000
numbers will decline slightly, but increases will occur amongst the most-

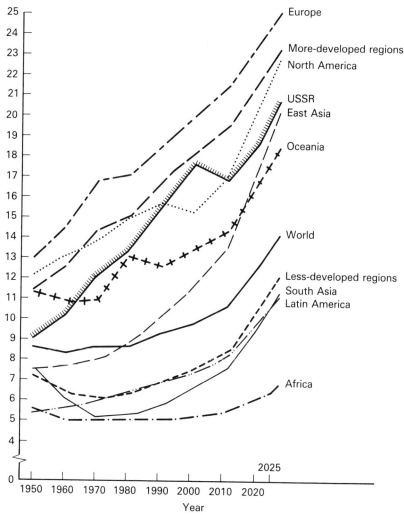

Figure 2.2 Percentage of total population 60 years and over: projection (Siegel and Hoover, 1982; reproduced with permission of WHO)

elderly people, that is the 74–84 age group and the 85-plus age group, so the proportion of the 'young old' and the 'old old' will change (see Fig. 2.3). Although there will be fewer elderly people in the year 2000, the numbers of very elderly people will be larger. This of course means a relative increase in the frail and the probability is that there will be more need for health and social services. It has recently been shown that it is the over 75 year age group that has the highest level of disability (OPCS, 1988). The effect will be a disability explosion. The people born in the post war 'baby boom' will start to retire around 2010 and the number of 'young olds' will start to increase again at that time.

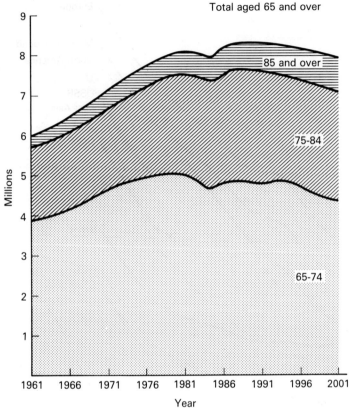

Figure 2.3 Future predictions

REFERENCES

DHSS (1983) *Command paper 8173: Growing Older*, HMSO, London.
Grundy, E. (1983) Demography and old age. *Journal of the American Geriatrics Society*, **31**, (6), 325–32.
OPCS (1975) *Census 1971: Great Britain – Household Composition, Summary Tables*, HMSO, London.
OPCS (1983a) *Census 1981: Persons of Pensionable Age*, HMSO, London.
OPCS (1983b) *Census 1981: National Report Great Britain – Part I*, HMSO, London.
OPCS (1988). *Surveys of disability in Great Britain. Report 1. The prevalence of disability among adults.* HMSO, London.
OPCS *Registrar General's Decennial Censuses of England and Wales 1851–1981*, HMSO, London.
Siegel, J. S. and Hoover, S. L. (1982) Demographic aspects of the health of the elderly to the year 2000 and beyond. *World Health Statistics Quarterly*, 35, 3/4, pp. 133–202.
Smith, C. (1988) Personal communication.
Smith, C. and Ebrahim, S. (1984) Number of centenarians. *Br. Med. J.*, **1288**, 772.

3 Health status

Although there is a general feeling that health status of individuals aged 65 and over is improving gradually and the general health of the elderly population is good, it is difficult to produce clear evidence of this. Mortality statistics are sometimes used as a guide but it is important to recognize that health is not reflected by levels of mortality. Nonetheless it is interesting to observe the trend. Total deaths registered in 1986 for England and Wales were 581 203, a decrease of 1.6% over the 1985 figure. The crude death rate was 11.6 per thousand population, compared with 11.8 for 1985, indicating that the decline that has taken place in recent years has been continued. Analysed by age, most of the reduction in 1986 was in the age range 45–64. Overall there was a fall in deaths due to diseases of the circulatory system of 3% and of the respiratory system of 2%. Examination of the crude death rates of the over-65 age group in this year shows that there has been little recent change. In this group the dominant cause of death was heart disease, followed closely by respiratory disease. The five most common causes of death in the 60–84-year age group for men and women are shown in Table 3.1. Figure 3.1 shows the relative changes in the proportions as age advances. Death from cancer becomes proportionately less in the older age groups. It is clear that an effective preventive programme targeted at ischaemic heart disease and cerebrovascular disease could change the mortality statistics dramatically. Studies aimed to demonstrate the effects of such initiatives, especially in primary care, need to be undertaken urgently.

Considering morbidity, the three National Morbidity Studies carried out in general practice over the past three decades have turned out to be unhelpful in assessing health status in elderly people. The rates of patients consulting per 1000 at risk in the over-65 age groups are seen in Table 3.2. This shows an increase in overall consultation levels for both men and women in 1981/82 compared with 1971/72. This increase applies particularly to the over-65 age group. The General Household Survey (1982) (OPCS, 1984) gives details of patients consulting a GP in the fourteen days before interview (see Table 3.3). The levels of consultation clearly increase with age and in the over-75 age group reached levels only slightly less than in the 0–4 age group.

There has been a tendency to treat elderly people as a homogeneous

Table 3.1 Five main causes of death at age 60–84 (and percentages of all causes of deaths) by sex, England, 1984

	Males		Females	
	Cause	(%)	Cause	(%)
1	Ischaemic heart disease	33	Ischaemic heart disease	27
2	Malignant neoplasm of respiratory and intrathoracic organs	11	Cerebrovascular disease	16
3	Cerebrovascular disease	10	Malignant neoplasm of digestive organs and peritoneum	8
4	Malignant neoplasm of digestive organs and peritoneum	8	Malignant neoplasm of bone, connective tissue, skin and breast	5
5	Chronic obstructive pulmonary disease	8	Malignant neoplasm of respiratory and intrathoracic organs	4
	Remainder	30		40

Source: Alderson and Ashwood (1985)

Table 3.2 Patients consulting: rates per 1000 persons at risk by age group and sex, 1955/6, 1971/2, 1981/2

Year	Sex	All ages	65–74	65 and over	75 and over
1955/6	M	630		680	
	F	700		730	
1971/2	M	622	645		663
	F	700	661		662
1981/2	M	652	721		777
	F	766	753		795

Source: OPCS (1986)

Table 3.3 Average number of consultations per person per year (Great Britain 1982)

Age	Male	Female	Total
0–4	7.2	6.4	6.8
5–15	3.0	3.0	3.0
16–44	2.2	5.2	3.7
45–64	4.1	5.1	4.6
65–74	4.9	5.5	5.3
75 and over	6.3	6.0	6.1

Source: OPCS (1984)

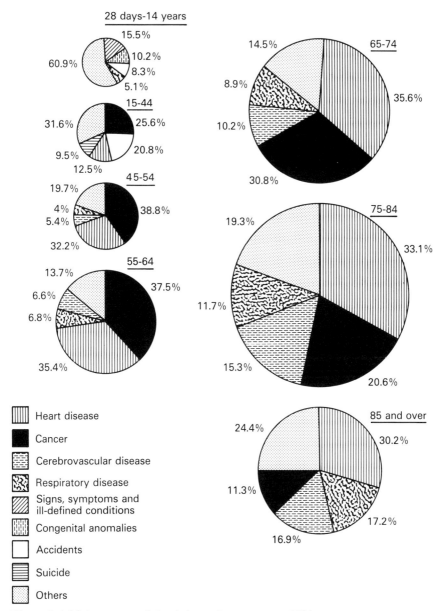

Figure 3.1 Main causes of death in each age group, 1986
Source: OPCS (1987)

group with regard to health status, but it is now clear that there are changes as age advances, although it is not possible to identify age 'cut-off' points neatly as a considerable variation exists in all age bands. It is possible to see differences between the 'young old' (65–74) and the 'old

old' (over 75). Those over 75 tend to have more longstanding health problems, they experience more illnesses and their use of services increases. Taylor and Ford (1983) examining age cohorts in a random sample of elderly persons in the community found evidence of these age changes. Using the number of chronic conditions present, symptoms experienced, and difficulties in functioning as three objective indices, they found that health advantage lay with the younger rather than the older cohort, males over females and the middle class over the working class. This general pattern of advantage was also found to be present in the fourth index studied, which was subjective self-ratings.

There have also been epidemiological health studies of elderly people. Audrey Hunt (1978) studying over-65-year-old people, found evidence that real physical old age, in the sense that it is generally understood, does not begin at 65 years for the majority. Most people between the ages of 65 and 75 were able to go about without assistance, were in reasonable health and enjoyed hobbies, interests and social contacts. Nevertheless, as age advanced, Hunt found that changes did occur in the 75–84 age group. A measurable decline was found in mobility, health and ability to perform personal and domestic tasks.

Many 'case finding' or screening studies have been carried out in populations of old persons (Williamson et al., 1964; Williams et al., 1972; Currie et al., 1974). These have often been based in general practice. Problems have been identified and some of these were previously unknown to the primary-care teams. This phenomenon persists. Vetter, Jones and Victor (1986) recruited a random sample of patients aged 70 years or over from the practice list of a general practice and allocated these patients to a health visitor for two years. The health visitor was instructed to give a major check-up annually to all her patients. The group consisted of 253 in the first year and 243 in the second. In the first year's assessment, only 21 individuals had no difficulties, whereas a total of 774 individual problems were identified in the remainder of the study group. These included physical, mental, social, environmental and carer problems. Of the physical conditions, the most common were those attributable to the cardiovascular system, followed by joint problems, eyesight defects and trouble with feet. The majority, but not all, of the physical and mental problems were known to the doctor. The report makes the point that the problems uncovered by the health visitor were not trivial and that a further assessment of the same subjects after one year continued to reveal more problems.

Precise morbidity levels in an elderly population are therefore not easy to define and the use of services and consultation rates may not be good indications. Morbidity may be unreported and not recognized. The patterns of morbidity may also change with time and it cannot be assumed that levels will remain constant. Probably a more important assessment is the functional ability of an elderly population. In 1972 Williams introduced a concept of effective health based on activities of daily living. Three groups were identified:

Group 1 Patients who were able to do their own cooking, housework and shopping, had cheerful and normal mental state and no incapacitating illness;

Group 2 Patients whose movements were restricted, often housefast, unable to do their own shopping, but were able to cook and do some housework. Mental deterioration may be present but they were coping with the situation. These patients often had illnesses but were able to manage to deal with their problems;

Group 3 These were usually bedfast patients. They were unable to cook, do their housework or shopping. There was often general restriction of movements. They may have had mental deterioration or incapacitating illness.

He found in a practice cohort of patients over the age of 75 years that 60% were in Group 1, 36% in Group 2 and 4% in Group 3.

Clarke (1984) assessed by interview the health and social status of old people over the age of 75 in Melton Mowbray, Leicestershire. He measured functional ability by using activities of daily living. A high proportion was able to perform personal tasks independently (see Table 3.4). As Clarke *et al.* pointed out, it was remarkable that, given help, almost the entire sample was able to perform all the listed activities.

Luker and Perkins (1987) provide additional evidence for an optimistic view of the health status of elderly people. They found that over 90% of elderly people questioned in a survey they undertook in Manchester

Table 3.4 Activities of daily living: independence, uses help, uses aids. Patients over 75

Activity	*Independent* (%)	*Uses aids* (%)	*Uses help* (%)	*Uses aids and help* (%)	*Not tested* (%)
Bathing	64.0	18.8	11.3	5.5	0.4
Able to get to and from toilet at night	68.2	29.9	0.3	1.2	0.4
Able to get around dwelling	81.1	17.0	0.7	0.6	0.7
Able to get in and out of chair	89.7	8.1	1.3	0.5	0.5
Able to get in and out of bed	93.0	3.2	2.8	0.8	0.1
Able to dress	93.8	0.9	4.6	0	0.6

Source: Clarke (1984)

rated their health as being fair to good. Over 80% of their sample were able to use public transport and only a minority required assistance to get around. Freer (1988) points out that there are important differences between recent studies and earlier screening surveys. The latter set out to identify problems and detect asymptomatic deviations from the norm. The former, on the other hand, have tried to assess the functional implications of the problem. Freer further points out that recent studies have tended to include the individual's rating of his/her own health. It is clearly important to understand how older people see themselves and not to rely on the expectations and beliefs of younger people about health status in old age.

REFERENCES

Alderson, M. and Ashwood, F. (1985) Projection of mortality rates for the elderly. *Population Trends*, **43**, 22–9, HMSO.

Clarke, M.E. (1984) Problems of the elderly: an epidemiological perspective. *J.R. Coll. Gen. Pract.*, **18** (2), 128.

Currie, G. MacNeill, R.M., Walker, J.G. *et al.* (1974) Medical and social screening of patients aged 70 to 72 by an urban general practice health team. *Br. Med. J.*, **2**, 108–11.

Freer, C. (1988) Old myths: frequent misconceptions about the elderly, in *The Ageing Population: Burden or Challenge?* (eds. N. Wells and C. Freer) Macmillan, London, Chapter 1.

Hunt, A. (1978) *The Elderly at Home*, Office of Population Censuses and Surveys, Social Services Division, HMSO, London.

Luker, K. and Perkins, E. (1987) The elderly at home: service needs and provisions. *J. R. Coll. Gen. Pract.*, **37**, 248.

OPCS (1984) *General Household Survey 1982*, HMSO, London.

OPCS (1986) Third national study of morbidity statistics from general practice 1981/2. *OPCS Monitor Ref. MB5 86/1*. January.

OPCS (1987) Deaths by cause, 1986. *OPCS Monitor* Ref. DH2 87/3. September.

Taylor, R.C. and Ford, G.G. (1983) Inequalities in old age. *Ageing and Society*, **3**, pt. 2, 183–208.

Vetter, N.J., Jones, D.A. and Victor, C.R. (1986) A health visitor affects the problems others do not reach. *Lancet* **ii**, 30.

Williams, E.I., Bennet, F.M., Nixon, J.V. *et al.* (1972) A socio-medical study of patients over 75 in general practice. *Br. Med. J.*, **2**, 445–8.

Williamson, J., Stokoe, I.H., Gray, S. *et al.* (1964) Old people at home. Their unreported needs. *Lancet* **i**, 1117–20.

4 *Social status*

In the United Kingdom information exists about the social status of old people, and from it a picture can be gained about how they live in the community. It has been possible to discern changes over the past two decades and the trends are often relevant to care provisions.

ELDERLY PEOPLE LIVING ALONE

Estimates of the number of old persons living alone vary, but the level is probably increasing and is higher in the older age groups. There are, however, differences in definition between various surveys and censuses that have made it difficult to obtain accurate assessments. The 1981 census gave details of the number of private households with one elderly resident as a proportion of all households. An analysis of these findings by age is given in Fig. 4.1. The 14.2% of all households that had as head an elderly single person gives an impression of the size of this group. Audrey Hunt, in 1978, found that nearly 30% of persons over 65 years old are living alone as are 21% of over-65-year-old men. The proportion of elderly men living alone almost doubled between 1959 and 1982, that is undertaken. Abrams (1983) states that nearly half of women over 65 years old are living alone as are 21% of over-65-year-old men. The proportion of elderly men living alone almost doubled between 1959 and 1982, that is from 11% to 21%. The main characteristic of elderly men was, however, that over 60% of them still share their dwelling with one other person, usually a wife, who was, on average, about three years younger than her husband.

Living alone does not of course always mean social isolation, that is without contact with neighbours and relatives. In fact the reverse is often true, particularly if an old person has lived in the same area for most of his or her life. Many old people live alone by choice and although acceptance of a measure of loneliness is necessary, they nevertheless enjoy an active social life. A distinction, therefore, has to be made between those living alone and the section within this main group who may be called 'isolates'. These are people who do not have any contact with friends or relatives and may often be found in a miserable and neglected state. The main members of this group are the unmarried and those who never had

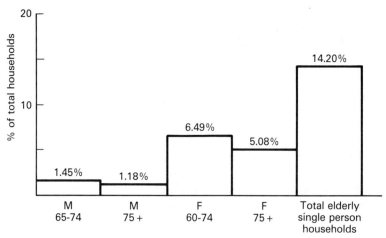

Figure 4.1 Private households with only one resident (elderly) as a proportion of all households, Great Britain 1981 (OPCS, 1983a)

children. There is also more risk of elderly persons being socially isolated if they had sons and not daughters. Young men are more easily drawn into their wives' families and may lose contact with their own parents. Fathers tend to have weaker ties with children and old men living alone are very liable to have no contact with their offspring. This, however, may be a class-related phenomenon and middle-class sons do tend to have stronger ties with their fathers.

Loneliness, on the other hand, is a different type of experience and this may happen even if an old person is living with a large family. By contrast, some who live in extreme isolation maintain that they are never lonely and obviously have inner resources to help them. This is helped by the previous life style and if letter writing or telephone communication has been the habit, communications are maintained. There are, however, special situations that help to produce social isolation and these will be discussed later in the chapter on social vulnerability. People living alone are subject to many hazards, one of which is poor nutrition, which can lead to deficiency.

FAMILY STRUCTURE OF THOSE NOT LIVING ALONE

Audrey Hunt (1978) gives information as to the family structure of old people and this can be seen in Table 4.1. As expected, husband and wife living together in a one-generation household is the most common pattern. It might be presumed that these couples manage their own domestic affairs but there is evidence from other surveys, for instance that of Gruer (1975), to suggest that much help is also forthcoming from

Table 4.1 Type of household in which elderly people live (from a survey of a sample of 1975 households in England)

	Men and women				Men				Women			
	Total	65–74	Age 75–84	85+	All men	65–74	Age 75–84	85+	All women	65–74	Age 75–84	85+
All elderly persons:												
(weighted)	3869	2571	1089	209	1540	1101	384	55	2329	1470	705	254
(unweighted figures)	2622	1354	1063	205	994	565	375	54	1628	789	688	151
Type of household	%	%	%	%	%	%	%	%	%	%	%	%
1. One elderly person alone	29.6	25.0	37.4	44.0	15.6	13.6	19.8	27.3	38.8	33.6	47.1	50.0
2. One elderly person with non-elderly spouse only	7.4	10.4	1.7	–	15.8	20.5	4.4	–	1.9	2.9	0.3	–
3. One elderly person with next generation only	6.7	4.3	10.6	17.2	2.9	2.0	4.2	10.9	9.3	6.0	14.0	19.5
4. One elderly person, non-elderly spouse and next generation only	1.7	2.4	0.3	–	4.2	5.6	0.8	–	–	–	–	–
5. One elderly person with others	5.9	5.6	6.4	7.7	4.7	4.2	6.0	7.2	6.7	6.7	6.7	7.7
6. Elderly married couple only	36.7	40.2	33.1	11.5	46.0	43.5	55.5	30.9	30.4	37.8	20.9	4.5
7. Elderly siblings only	2.8	2.3	3.9	2.9	1.0	0.8	1.0	5.5	4.0	3.4	5.5	1.9
8. Elderly married couple with next generation only	4.1	5.1	2.3	1.4	5.1	5.5	4.2	3.6	3.4	4.7	1.3	0.6
9. Other combinations of two or more elderly persons with others	5.1	4.7	4.2	15.3	4.5	4.2	4.2	14.5	5.5	5.0	4.3	15.6
Total	100.0	100.0	100.0	100.0	100.0	100.0	100.0	100.0	100.0	100.0	100.0	100.0

Source: Hunt (1978)

relatives and friends in these circumstances and few of these old people are obliged to be self-sufficient. The Gruer survey was undertaken in the Scottish Borders and the high level of help available might reflect the basically rural character of the region. The reason for living in a one-generation household was sometimes because the old people had no children, and when this was the case there was evidence that domestic co-operation occurred between brothers and sisters of the same generation. The level of support that two old people, whether married or siblings, can give each other is quite remarkable and despite frailty they manage to cope with their own domestic problems.

A sizeable minority of old people live in a two-generation home. This is where a house is shared with children, either married or unmarried. The two-generation households sometimes require considerable role adjustment by the members, particularly the two women. When the shared house is the original family home, the mother's authority is usually maintained, but where a daughter-in-law is involved, friction may easily occur and there is danger of the elderly woman becoming a subordinate housekeeper. Harmony can only be preserved by responsibilities being carefully defined. This is one reason why old people prefer to live alone. It is easier when married children live with old parents because the old mother retains her original role, but this can be affected by her state of health. It is easier for an old person to reciprocate services when there are grandchildren to look after and babysitting is necessary. The number of three-generation households is, however, diminishing. In 1959 only 8% of elderly women lived in a household that contained a child under the age of 15; and by 1982, even this small proportion had fallen to 2% for both men and women (Abrams, 1983). This undoubtedly is due to the desire of young people to create an independent home away from their parents and their increasing economic ability to do so. Old people may also want to live alone and value their privacy especially when the house, as is becoming more likely, is small.

AREAS OF RESIDENCE

Contemporary ageing has produced an interesting and distinctive geography of elderly people. This has taken the form of retirement migration to coastal areas, particularly in the South-East, which has produced the so-called 'Costa Geriatrica'. In the United States of America, Florida is similarly a receiving state for such migration. The movement is usually from urban areas. Broxtowe, an urban area in Nottinghamshire, has 14% over-65-year-olds, 5% over-75-year olds and nearly 1% over-85-year olds, compared with Worthing in Sussex, which has 31% over-65-year olds, 14% over-75-year olds and nearly 4% over-85-year olds. The presence of the sea makes the difference. The pattern is true in other regions that involve coastal resorts. In 1971 Grange in Lancashire had 45% elderly persons, Sidmouth in Devon 44% and Colwyn Bay in North Wales 32%. Reasons for this migration include the wider take-up of retirement at 65, better pension provisions and greater opportunities for movement and travel. The increased migration of younger members of a family has frequently meant that there are no family reasons for parents and grandparents to stay in the family home and they are free to move to what they see to be more congenial surroundings. It is likely that these patterns of migration will continue unless saturation of retirement areas deters further movement. As economic circumstances change, however, it is just possible that staying in the same area during retirement may become more popular and the advantages may be realized of staying in a pre-established household amongst old friends and neighbours.

The other place where there are concentrations of elderly people is in the inner cities. The reasons are twofold: migration of younger people out of the poorer areas once they have enough capital to acquire better quality suburban housing, and the fact that many elderly people may not wish to leave the inner-city house in which they have spent most of their lives. They also may not be able to afford the move. This is very clearly illustrated in the distribution of the elderly in Wichita, Kansas, USA (see Fig. 4.2). It is a good example of what is likely to be happening in any city in the Western world.

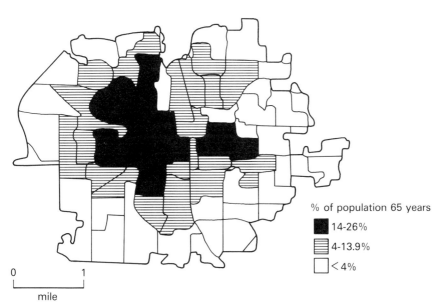

% of population 65 years

■ 14-26%

▤ 4-13.9%

□ < 4%

0   1

mile

Figure 4.2 Distribution of elderly in Wichita, Kansas, USA (Cowgill and Ostertag, 1962)

TYPE OF HOUSEHOLD TENURE

There were almost 19.5 million households in Great Britain at the time of the 1981 census. Of these, nearly 7 million had one or more persons of pensionable age; half were owner-occupied and over one-third council-rented (see Table 4.2). The general trend is towards more owner-occupied houses and this also applies to elderly people. The number of elderly people in owner-occupied households rose from 44% in 1959 to 52% in 1982 (Abrams, 1983).

Table 4.2 Tenure of households with one or more persons of pensionable age (Great Britain)

All households with one or more persons of pensionable age*	Number 6 765 886	% 100
Owner-occupied	3 430 227	50.7
Rented from council	2 404 014	35.5
Rented from Housing Association	173 535	2.6
Rented with business	13 800	0.2
Rented by virtue of employment	40 067	0.6
Other rented: unfurnished	639 806	9.5
Other rented: furnished	64 437	1.0

* There were a total of 19 411 566 households in Great Britain at the time of the 1981 census

Source: OPCS (1983b)

HOUSEHOLD AMENITIES AND TRANSPORT

Elderly persons have also shared the increase in the ownership of consumer goods seen in the general population. Abrams states that in 1982 36% of over-65-year olds lived in a household with a car and two-thirds of them in a household with a telephone (see Table 4.3). These figures may, however, mask some important regional variations.

The transport situation is even more complicated because the possession of a car in a household changes with age. This can be seen when considering the number of households that have no car.

39% of all British households have no car;
62% of households with one or more persons of pensionable age have no car;
69% of households with a lone man aged 65–74 years have no car;
83% of households with a lone man aged 75 and over have no car;
86% of households with a lone woman aged 60–74 have no car;
95% of households with a lone woman aged 75 and over have no car.

(Source: OPCS, 1983b)

Table 4.3 Possession of consumer goods, 1959 and 1982, Great Britain

% of people living in households with:	Aged 65 or over		All aged 15 or over	
	1959	1982	1959	1982
Washing machine	22	70	38	84
Car	16	36	28	66
Refrigerator	12	88	24	93
Telephone	9	64	22	74
Television:				
BBC only	13	0	12	0
BBC and ITV	42	96	63	99

Source: Abrams (1983) (reproduced with permission of HMSO)

Older persons are therefore very dependent upon others for transport and this can cause difficulties.

There are also problems with public transport. A short series of questions was included in the 1982 General Household Survey (OPCS, 1984) about travel by bus. Overall, 62% of the informants aged 16 and over had used a local bus in the six months prior to the interview, although there was some variation according to age. The proportion was highest (83%) amongst those aged between 16 and 19. It fell to 53% amongst the age group 30–44 years and then rose again to over 70% amongst older informants. The proportion using buses fell steeply over the age of 80. Under the age of 75, women were much more likely than men to use buses, but the difference was reversed amongst very elderly people. Women aged 70 and over were much more likely than men of comparable age to say they had difficulty with buses.

One-tenth of all bus users said that there was something about their general health that made using buses difficult for them, the most common difficulty being getting on and off the bus. This was experienced by 25% of the group of bus users aged 75 years and over. The proportion of cases having physical difficulty increased markedly with age and was up to 33% of those aged 75 and over (OPCS, 1984).

PETS AND HOBBIES

In common with the rest of the population, pet ownership is becoming less popular with elderly people. In 1959, 42% of all elderly people had at least one pet. In 1981–2 the figure had fallen to 33%, with only dogs retaining their 1959 popularity at 18% (men) and 16% (women) (Abrams, 1983).

The Abrams study also revealed that about one half of the elderly (over 65) population had holidays, either in the UK or abroad. There has been little difference in the pattern since 1959. Almost all elderly persons have a colour television. Cinema going has fallen amongst elderly people to no more than 7% in 1982. The non-smokers increased from 62% in 1959 to 73% in 1982. Pipe-smoking has declined from 10% to 3% in that time. On the other hand, consumption of alcohol has remained popular, and, if anything, increased in elderly people. For men in 1959, the percentage for beer drinking was 70%, wine drinking 53% and spirit drinking 58%. In 1981–2 the proportions were 76%, 53% and 77% respectively.

WORK/EMPLOYMENT

There have been important changes in the pattern of employment of over-65-year olds over the past ten years. The percentage of men aged 55 and over who remain economically active has declined steadily since 1973. By 1984 under three-quarters of men aged between 55 and 59 were working and only half of those aged 60 to 64. This decline reflects the trend towards earlier retirement. Over the same period, the proportion of men over 65 in employment fell from 19% to 9%. The number of women economically active over the age of 65 has always been relatively low. In 1984 the level was 3%. By this time, however, a sizeable minority of women who were retired workers enjoying pensions had developed. Most men and women are therefore retired by the time they reach 65. It is also true that those who remain economically active are mainly part-time workers.

HOSPITAL IN-PATIENT LEVEL

The numbers of persons of all ages admitted to hospital in England and Wales in 1984 was over 5 million, including those with mental illness and mental handicap. The over-65 age group contributed well over a million and a half to this total. In the 65–74 age group the sex ratio was about equal but in the over-75 age group there were many more women (see Table 4.4). Although the average number of in-patient stays per 100 persons per year between 1982 and 1984 was unchanged for the general population, there is evidence of increased use of in-patient beds by the very old. In the over-75 age group there was an increase from 19 to 22 per hundred persons for men and 17 to 20 per hundred persons for women (DHSS and OPCS, 1986). Between 1973 and 1983, all admissions for dementia doubled in England. The changing pattern of hospital in-patient usage is indicated by the 45% increase in the admission rate for the over 65s to mental illness hospitals in England and Wales between 1973 and 1983. The increase in the rate of first admission was only marginal (Smith, Staley and Arie, 1986).

Table 4.4 Hospital-patient activity: distribution by age group and sex – England 1984 – thousands

	All ages total	Under 5	5–14	15–19	20–24	25–34	35–44	45–54	55–64	65–74	75 and over
Persons: Total											
Mental illness*	192.3	0.2	1.7	5.5	13.0	29.8	30.9	24.8	25.7	25.3	35.5
Mental handicap*	35.0	1.1	9.6	8.2	5.7	5.6	2.4	1.3	0.7	0.3	0.1
Non-psychiatric†	4947.7	421.6	374.8	243.6	279.7	492.2	477.5	470.0	620.0	710.6	857.7
Male: Total											
Mental illness*	80.3	0.1	1.0	2.7	6.9	15.1	14.5	10.4	9.7	9.0	10.8
Mental handicap*	19.3	0.7	5.7	4.4	3.2	3.0	1.1	0.7	0.3	0.1	–
Non-psychiatric†	2321.9	252.5	222.2	109.4	113.3	175.5	179.9	217.7	341.3	373.9	336.2
Female: Total											
Mental illness*	111.9	0.1	0.7	2.8	6.0	14.7	16.4	14.4	15.9	16.2	24.7
Mental handicap*	15.7	0.4	3.9	3.7	2.5	2.6	1.3	0.7	0.4	0.1	0.1
Non-psychiatric†	2625.8	169.1	152.6	134.2	166.4	316.7	297.6	252.3	278.7	336.7	521.5

* Figures for psychiatric hospitals and units are in terms of admissions because a small proportion of their patients stay for relatively long periods and admissions give a better indication of the current activity.

† Figures for non-psychiatric hospitals are in terms of discharges and include deaths in hospitals. Persons treated in the obstetric and GP maternity specialties are excluded. Private patients are included in the data.

Source: DHSS and OPCS (1986)

PRIVATE NURSING HOMES, REST HOMES AND
LOCAL AUTHORITY ACCOMMODATION

Data on the number of beds for elderly people in private nursing homes
is sparse. Recent figures obtained from the DHSS suggest a rapid increase
(see Table 4.5). The number of beds almost doubled between 1982 and
1985.

Table 4.5 Private nursing homes in England

Date	Beds for the elderly	Number of institutions
1985 (December)	33 012	1633
1984 (December)	26 507	1296
1983 (December)	21 622	1127
1982 (December)	17 728	1036

Source: DHSS Personal Communication (1988)

On the other hand, persons in accommodation provided by or on behalf
of local authorities for the elderly or younger physically handicapped
persons have changed very little since 1980 (see Table 4.6). The number of
voluntary homes has not increased since 1980 but the number of private
rest homes has increased dramatically (see Chapter 9). There are regional
variations in the provision of non-hospital beds for elderly people.
Broadly, public provision by local authorities is highest in the North and

Table 4.6 Persons in accommodation provided by or on behalf of local authorities
for the elderly or younger physically handicapped (England)*

		1975	1980[†]	1981	1982	1983	1984	1985[‡]
Persons provided	T	119 997	128 134	126 990	125 974	124 562	120 890	118 051
with accommodation	M	35 923	35 441	34 762	34 623	33 102	31 690	30 683
	F	84 074	92 693	92 228	91 351	91 460	89 200	87 368
Aged under 65	T	10 254	9 321	9 782	9 129	8 924	8 687	8 046
	M	5 173	4 700	4 955	4 700	4 532	4 482	4 113
	F	5 081	4 621	4 827	4 429	4 392	4 205	3 933
Aged 65 and over	T	109 743	118 813	117 208	116 845	115 538	112 203	110 005
	M	30 750	30 741	29 807	29 923	28 470	27 208	26 570
	F	78 993	88 072	87 401	86 922	87 068	84 995	83 435
Number of homes[§]		2 459	2 638	2 658	2 662	2 669	2 673	–

* Accommodation provided under Sections 21(1)(a) and 26(1)(a) of *the National Assistance
Act* 1948. Prior to 1976 figures excluded short–stay residents.
[†] From 1980 short–stay homes are included.
[‡] From 1985 data were also collected on residents in unregistered premises with less than 4
places. These are excluded from the above table.
[§] Excluding voluntary or private homes.

Source: DHSS and OPCS (1986)

lowest in the South, with the Midlands being in the middle range. Conversely, voluntary, especially private provisions, are highest in the South and lowest in the North. The North/South divide is attributable to the greater wealth of the southern part of Britain and in addition the large concentration of elderly persons on the South-East coast. Despite these increases, however, the overwhelming majority of elderly people live in private households. On census night in 1981, 95.3% of the pensionable population in Great Britain was in a private household (OPCS, 1983b).

REFERENCES

Abrams, M. (1983) Changes in the lifestyles of the elderly 1959–1982. *Social Trends*, **14**, 11–16.

Cowgill, D.O. and Ostertag, S.F. (1962) The people of Wichita, 1960. The Urban Studies Centre, Wichita, Kansas.

DHSS and OPCS (1986) *Health and Personal Social Services Statistics for England*, HMSO, London.

Gruer, R. (1975) *Needs of the Elderly in the Scottish Borders*, Scottish Home and Health Department, Edinburgh.

Hunt, A. (1978) *The Elderly at Home*, Office of Population Censuses and Surveys, Social Survey Division, HMSO, London.

OPCS (1983a) *Census 1981: National Report Great Britain – Part II*, HMSO London.

OPCS (1983b) *Census 1981: Persons of Pensionable Age*, HMSO, London.

OPCS (1984) *General Household Survey 1982*, HMSO, London.

OPCS (1987) *Deaths by cause, 1986*. OPCS Monitor, Ref. DH2 87/3.

Smith, C.W., Staley, C.J. and Arie, T. (1986) Admission of demented old people to psychiatric units: an assessment of recent trends. *Br. Med. J.*, **292**, 731.

5 Economic status

Retirement marks the point when most people stop earning and come to depend upon pensions and benefits, either from the State or private schemes to which they have been contributing during their working lives. They also, to some extent, depend upon their savings. In assessing the economic position of pensioners, it is necessary to take account of these aspects and also the changes that have occurred both in the actual levels of economic provision and how these have changed relative to non-pensioners.

DISPOSABLE INCOME

There are problems in calculating disposable income that result in conflicting data. Two recent papers give details: Abrams (1983) and Fiegehen (1986). Fiegehen gives information that covers everyone over pensionable age. Abrams, on the other hand, refers to a subset of persons in what he terms 'special pensioner households' who had at least 75% of their income from National Insurance, retirement or similar pension and/or supplementary pension. There are other complicated differences in the way in which the economic status of elderly persons is presented and this makes it difficult to make broad generalizations about disposable incomes. The overall figures inevitably hide the plight of subgroups who, for one reason or another, are disadvantaged.

However, the figures quoted by Fiegehen do give an idea of the trends. The calculated disposable income of pensioners is made up of all income, including investment, savings, pensions and other social-security benefits. It is a net figure representing the spending power, after deductions for income tax, National Insurance and occupational pension contributions. These deductions are relatively low amongst pensioners.

Pensioners' share of overall total personal disposable income has more than doubled since 1951 (see Table 5.1). This reflects the growth of the number of pensioners as well as rising incomes. When measured in real terms, allowing for price rises, pensioners' disposable income per head has nearly tripled since 1951, compared with an increase of only two-thirds for people below pensionable age. Although always likely to change, pensioners' disposable income is now about 70% of that

Table 5.1 Growth of pensioners' incomes (Great Britain) (all figures are percentages)

	Total population	Pensioners' share of		Growth in real disposable income per head in previous 10 years		Pensioners' disposable income per head relative to non-pensioners
		Total adult population	Total personal disposable income	Pensioners	Non-pensioners	
1951	13.5	17.5	7	–	–	41
1961	14.5	19	8.5	48	31	47
1971	16.5	21.5	11.5	42	16	57
1981–2	17.5	23	14.5	31	10	68
1984–5*	18	23	15	–	–	69

* Projections

Source: Fiegehen (1986) (reproduced with permission of HMSO)

Table 5.2 Main components of pensioners' total income, Great Britain

	NI retirement pension	Other social security benefits*	Total income from the state	Occupational pensions	Earnings	Investment income	Total gross income	Income tax and NI contributions[†]
Percentage of total gross income								
1951	35	8	42	15	27	15	100	12
1961	41	6	48	16	22	15	100	10
1971	40	7	48	21	18	13	100	11
1981–2	47	12	59	21	10	10	100	11
1984–5[‡]	49	11	60	22	9	9	100	11

* Mainly supplementary and housing benefit. Growth in the 1970s was largely due to housing and disability benefits.
[†] NI contributions were paid by workers over pension age until 1978.
[‡] Projections.

Source: Fiegehen (1986) (reproduced with permission of HMSO)

of non-pensioners. The main source of the improvement is the growing value of National Insurance basic pension, compared with average take-home pay.

In answer to a Parliamentary question on 9 February 1988 Mr Nicholas Scott stated that a pensioner's income grew on average by 2.7% a year in real terms between 1979 and 1985: 18% over the whole period. This rate of increase was more than twice as fast as for the population as a whole. How much of this was due to state pension schemes and how much to private pension schemes was not stated.

The number of retirement pensioners increased by 9% between 1980 and 1986 and a further 1% increase was likely in 1987. Retirement pensions easily represent the largest single item of Social-Security expenditure.

The number of pensioners claiming what was then called 'National Assistance' rose steadily from 0.6 million in 1948 to 1.1 million in 1958. There was a sharp rise in numbers in 1968 as a result of the changeover to the Supplementary Benefit system in 1966. In spite of the increase in the numbers of pensioners since then, there has been a drop to 1.7 million claimants for Supplementary Benefit in 1984. This reflects improvements in the provision of retirement income, such as occupational schemes, and the introduction of Housing Benefit (HMSO, 1987).

The income derived from the state has risen as a proportion of pensioners' total gross income to about 60%. Occupational income has also risen but income from employment and investments has declined in relative importance (see Table 5.2). Although the general position of pensioners has improved considerably in the last thirty years, many pensioners still have low incomes. For most pensioners, the National Insurance basic pension is their largest single source of income and over one in five pensioners has income topped up by Supplementary Benefit, including one-third of widows (see Table 5.3). Two-thirds of pensioners received income from their own savings and investments, although often this was only a small proportion of their total income. An important additional asset for pensioners is their home, and half of pensioner households are owner-occupied.

HOW ELDERLY PEOPLE SPEND THEIR MONEY

Turning to Abrams' paper (1983), he considers the average weekly household expenditure between 1959 and 1981 and this is shown in Table 5.4. As mentioned earlier, the figures relate to special pensioner households in which at least three-quarters of the total income is derived from National Insurance retirement pension or similar pensions. The table shows comparisons between the proportion of average weekly expenditure on various items and how this has changed. It is interesting to see how an average pensioner family spends its money. Partly because

Table 5.3 Percentage of pensioners* supported by Supplementary Benefit: by age and sex, Great Britain, 1982

	Married couples[†]	Men	Non-married[‡] Women Widows	Other	Total
	(%)	*(%)*	*(%)*	*(%)*	*(%)*
Age groups					
60–64	–	–	23	27	25
65–69	9	20	33	28	15
70–74	14	21	42	31	23
75–79	17	28	43	27	28
80 or over	18	20	38	21	26
All of pension age	13	22	35	27	23

* People of state pension age.
† Classified by age of husband.
‡ Includes single, widowed, separated and divorced people.

Source: Fiegehen (1986) (reproduced with permission of HMSO)

of population changes the size of the average household declined from 3.08 persons to 2.73 persons over this period. This decline meant that although the weekly expenditure of the average UK household jumped from £15.50 to £125.41 (an eight-fold increase), weekly expenditure per capita in the average household rose from £5.03 to £45.96 (a nine-fold increase). Most of the extra spending merely reflected inflation. Between 1959 and 1981 the general index of retail prices registered a six-fold increase. However, even allowing for this inflation over the 22 years, real expenditure per capita of the average household still showed a substantial increase of 51%. If it is assumed that what happened to the disposable incomes and weekly expenditure of special pensioner households broadly reflected the experience of all pensioner households, then it appears that between 1959 and 1981 real per capita consumer spending in the average elderly household increased slightly less than in all households. Nevertheless, the increase was substantial.

BENEFIT ENTITLEMENT OF OLD PERSONS

In the years following World War II, a great number of welfare entitlements were made available to elderly people. Since the birth of the Welfare State, they have consistently been by far the largest group of consumers of benefits. Despite this, there is no doubt that many old people fail to claim all the benefits to which they are entitled. There are several reasons for this: the large number of benefits is confusing and there has been poor publicity in the past. Attitudes towards benefits

Table 5.4 Average weekly household expenditure, 1959 and 1981, United Kingdom

	All households		Special pensioner households		Expenditure of special pensioner households as a percentage of expenditure of all households	
	1959	1981	1959	1981	1959	1981
Average weekly household expenditure on (£s):						
Housing	1.45	19.76	0.91	10.52	63	53
Fuel, light and power	0.94	7.46	0.68	5.35	72	72
Food	5.01	27.20	1.98	13.35	40	49
Alcoholic drink	0.50	6.06	0.11	1.23	22	20
Tobacco	0.94	3.74	0.19	1.30	20	35
Clothing and footwear	1.58	9.23	0.34	2.38	22	26
Durable household goods	1.12	9.40	0.14	1.61	12	17
Other goods	1.11	9.45	0.35	3.03	31	32
Transport and vehicles	1.31	18.70	0.14	1.96	11	10
Services	1.46	13.84	0.33	4.06	23	29
Miscellaneous	0.06	0.58	–	0.08	1	14
Total household expenditure	15.50	125.41	5.16	44.86	33	36
Average weekly expenditure per person (£s)	5.03	45.96	3.71	32.32	74	70
Average number of people per household:						
Males	1.47	1.33	0.44	0.46		
Females	1.61	1.40	0.95	0.93		
Total	3.08	2.73	1.39	1.39		

Source: Family Expenditure Survey, 1959 and 1981 (From Abrams, 1983) (reproduced with permission of HMSO)

being charity and the pride that most old people take in being financially independent have deterred some from claiming. Again general practitioners, who are often the only source of advice to old people, have themselves been ignorant as to benefits and have sometimes been resistant to giving certificates of illness and disability. For this reason it is essential for health and social workers to have an idea of the benefits available. Unfortunately, these often change both in level and type, making it difficult to provide up-to-date information. In April 1988 changes were introduced in income-support benefits. The structure for the payment of basic retirement pension, additional pension, graduated pensions and over-eighties pension remain, however, unchanged. For details of actual payments involved it is necessary to consult up-to-date DSS information sheets. The basic broad categories can however be summarized.

Basic retirement pension

Providing they have satisfied National-Insurance contribution conditions and have retired from regular work, retirement pension, which is taxable, is paid to women over 60 and men over 65. Five years after these dates the basic pension is paid whether or not the individual is working. Retirement pension is paid to a married woman on her husband's contributions when he retires, providing that she is over 60 and has retired from regular work or has reached the age of 65. If a woman qualifies for a pension in her own right, as well as her husband's, she receives whichever pension is the higher. Four months before a man's sixty-fifth birthday and a woman's sixtieth birthday, the DSS sends out a form to allow individuals to claim their pension. Pensions are normally paid weekly by an order book, which is cashed at a post office, but pensions can be paid directly into a bank or building-society account as well as by book. For the housebound, a neighbour or relative can cash a pension on their behalf. The value of the pension is reviewed and usually increased yearly.

Additional pension

On 6 April 1978, the State Earnings-Related Pension scheme (SERPS) was started. This additional pension is based on earnings since April 1978. Where pensions are derived from state or employer superannuation schemes, the individual may be 'contracted out' of SERPS. Anyone not contracted out who retired after 6 April 1979 may qualify for an additional state pension, although as the scheme takes twenty years to reach maturity, no-one will receive a full additional pension until 1998. The additional pension is index-related to earnings from April 1978. Employees on a contracted-out pension scheme received a guaranteed minimum pension in place of the state additional pension.

Graduated pension

This is a taxable pension scheme that ended in April 1975, but those who received such a pension at that time still have it normally paid with the basic retirement pension. Anyone who paid graduated contributions will have this extra pension paid with their basic retirement pension when they retire. The amount of money received depends on how much was paid into the graduated scheme before 1975.

Over-eighties pension

This is a non-contributory retirement pension for people aged 80 and over who have no retirement pension arrangements or who have a retirement pension that is less than the amount payable to other pensioners. The pension is paid at a specific level per week, minus the value of any basic pension received.

Income Support

This has replaced Supplementary Benefit and supplementary-pension arrangements and came into force on 11 April 1988. It is a social-security benefit aimed at helping people who do not have enough money to live on. It is intended to meet regular weekly needs. People who were getting Supplementary Benefit and were entitled to Income Support will not normally get less money each week as a result of the change to Income Support. People who may get help from this benefit include people aged 60 and over and those staying at home to look after a disabled relative. People can get help from Income Support even if they have savings up to £8000. If someone who claims has a partner whom they are married to or live with as if they were married to them, they have their partner's savings counted as well. If the savings are worth up to £3000 it will make no difference to the Income Support they get. Savings between £3000 and £8000 will make a difference, each £250 or part of £250 will be treated as if it was bringing in £1 per week. There are personal allowances for day-to-day living expenses, which vary according to age and marital status. On top of this some people, for example, pensioners, the disabled and single parents, receive premiums. There are two rates of Pensioner Premium: one for single people and one for couples. There is also a Higher Pensioner Premium that can be given to anyone aged 80 or over or to a pensioner who is registered blind, or to a person aged between 60 and 79 who is getting Attendance or Mobility Allowance, Invalidity Benefit or Severe-Disablement Allowance. Normally only one of the premiums is paid – whichever is the higher. There is one other premium that a pensioner may get and that is the Severe Disability Premium. This is given when a person lives alone, receives Attendance Allowance and no-one is claiming Invalid-Care Allowance for them.

Social Fund

The Social Fund is a scheme to help people with exceptional expenses that are difficult for them to pay from regular income. Three types of discretionary payments have been introduced: Budgeting Loans, Crisis Loans and Community-Care Grants. There is a limited amount of money available for these payments. When applications are reviewed, Social-Fund officers have to take account of the needs of all people who apply for help and decide which needs can be met from the money available. Budgeting Loans are for people getting Income Support. They are to help them pay for something that is needed but cannot be afforded at the time. The loan needs to be paid back and this is done by taking money from the person's Social Security Benefit each week. Savings worth over £500 will make a difference to Budgeting Loans. A person applying for a Budgeting Loan, or their partner, must have been getting Income Support for each of the previous 26 weeks without a break, apart from the fact that one break of 14 days or less does not matter. People cannot get a Budgeting Loan if they or their partner are involved in a trade dispute and the Social-Fund officer must be sure that the person can afford to pay the money back. This will inevitably cause problems because it means that the really poor will probably be assessed as not having the ability to pay back, and yet it is probably just these who more than anyone else need to be given such a loan.

Crisis Loans are to help people to pay for things they need urgently because of an emergency or a disaster. Anyone may be able to get a Crisis Loan. They are not just for people getting Income Support or other Social Security Benefit. But people will only be able to get a Crisis Loan if there is no other way of preventing a serious risk to their health or safety, or that of their family. Someone may, for instance, get a Crisis Loan to pay for their immediate needs if they have been burgled or have no money or savings. Again, this Crisis Loan has to be paid back.

Community-Care Grants are for people getting Income Support and they are designed especially to help people return to the community after they have been in care. Being in care means having been in residence in hospitals, nursing homes, old people's homes and residential-care homes. It also can be applied to situations where a person needs help to stay in the community rather than having to be in care, or cope with very difficult problems in their family, such as disability, long-term illness or family breakdown. The grant can also be used to pay for fares to visit someone who is ill or for another urgent reason. If someone gets Income Support, they will not have to pay back Community-Care Grants. If someone does not get such support when they move into the community, they will have to pay back the grant. The Social-Fund officer will also give general financial help where someone appears to have budgeting difficulties.

Housing Benefit

Housing Benefit is a government scheme to help people on low incomes pay their rent and rates. It is run by local councils. Housing Benefit can be paid to people who are working or do not work, pay rent to a council or to a private landlord or own their home. People do not have to be getting other social security benefit. However, people with savings of more than £8000 cannot get Housing Benefit. Housing Benefit can cover some or all the rent and up to 80% of the rates that someone has to pay on their home. The benefit cannot normally help with the cost of buying a home, the cost of fuel for heating, lighting and cooking, the cost of meals that are included in the rent, water charges, some service charges for things like personal laundry and household cleaning, ground rent and service charges for homes if the lease was originally for more than 21 years. People who claim Income Support will normally be given a form for claiming Housing Benefit and the Social Security office will pass the form on to the local council to deal with. People who are not claiming Income Support and feel that they are entitled to Housing Benefit need to get such a form from their local council.

Invalidity Benefit

This is a tax-free benefit and is made up of Invalidity Pension and Invalidity Allowance. The pension replaces Statutory Sick Pay or Sickness Benefit after a person has been on this for 28 weeks. Invalidity Allowance is an extra allowance for people who first became incapable of work more than five years before state-pension age. Some people qualify for an earnings-related extra allowance instead of an age-related extra allowance. The rates depend on the age at which an individual was first unable to work. If illness begins after pensionable age, there is no Invalidity Benefit payable. This is probably unfair because it is likely to be at that point when it is most needed. However, Invalidity Benefit and Retirement Pension are the same amount of money so there is little advantage in being able to claim Invalidity Benefit after pension age. Anyone receiving Invalidity Benefit when they reach pension age can choose whether to take their Retirement Pension or stay on Invalidity Benefit for a further five years. The amount of benefit will not be any different, but Invalidity Benefit is not taxable income and Retirement Pension is.

Mobility Allowance

This benefit is designed to help the severely disabled become more mobile. It is a tax-free cash benefit for people aged between 5 and 75 who are unable or virtually unable to walk, but they have to qualify for the allowance before the age of 65 and they must apply before the age of 66. It is intended to help with the extra costs of getting about, but unfortunately it does not really include those who probably need it most, such as the over-75-year olds and those who only become eligible at the age of 66.

Attendance Allowance

Attendance Allowance is for people who are severely disabled, mentally or physically, and who require the attention of another person by day or by night for at least six months. There are two rates of payment: a lower rate for those requiring attention or supervision either by day or by night, and a higher rate, which is paid for those who require supervision for the whole twenty-four hours. Medical evidence is required and this means an examination by a doctor representing the DSS. Attendance Allowance is paid regardless of income, savings and National Insurance contributions and can be paid together with other benefits.

Invalid-Care Allowance

An Invalid-Care Allowance is available to any person who spends 35 hours per week or more looking after someone who is in receipt of an Attendance Allowance. The person claiming this must be under pension age.

Christmas Bonus

This tax-free bonus is automatically given during the week beginning 7 December to people receiving a Retirement Pension, Over-Eighties Pension, Widow's Pension, Attendance Allowance, Invalidity Pension, Severe Disablement Allowance, Supplementary Pension and Invalid-Care Allowance.

Widow's Benefits

Major changes in benefits for widows have been introduced since 11 April 1988. There are at present three main Widow's Benefits. They are Widow's Payment, Widowed Mother's Allowance and Widow's Pension. Usually women of pensionable age will not qualify for these benefits but there are some circumstances in which they may do so. The Widow's Payment is a tax-free lump sum payment of £1000 and is paid to widows who are under 60 or whose husbands were under 65 when they died. Widowed Mother's Allowance is a taxable weekly payment for widows who have dependent children until all the Child Benefit has stopped. Once Widowed Mother's Allowance stops, the widow would receive the Widow's Pension if she qualifies for that. Widow's Pension is a taxable weekly payment benefit paid to a widow who is 45 years or over when her husband dies or when Widowed Mother's Allowance ceases. All types of Widow's Benefits are paid only if the husband has paid National Insurance Contributions. A widow cannot receive any Widow's Benefit if she is divorced or not legally married or is living with another man as his wife.

Death Grant
The Social Fund is available to those people receiving Income Support, Housing Benefit or Family Credit. Any savings over £500 will reduce the amount of grant given.

Other allowances
There is also a variety of other allowances that are payable to older persons, which are dependent on special circumstances. Industrial Benefit was abolished on 11 April 1988 and is now only paid to those people who were receiving it before then. This is a short-term pension, the rate depending upon circumstances. Industrial Injuries Disablement Benefit is paid to a person who becomes disabled as the result of an accident at work or as the result of an industrial disease. Again the rate is dependent upon the severity of the disability. Sickness Benefit is paid to people who are unable to work because of sickness or disablement and is sometimes available over pension age where there is need to support children. War Disablement Pension is payable to people disabled as a result of service in the armed forces during the 1914–18 war or at any time after 2 September 1939. It is also paid to merchant seamen and civilians disabled during World War II. The amount depends upon the rank of the person and the severity of the disablement. War Widows or Dependant's Pension is also payable to relatives of a person who was killed in the armed forces or who died later as a result of injuries sustained in the armed forces. The amount paid depends upon the rank of the deceased, the age of the widow and the amount of other income and savings. Workman's Compensation Supplement is paid to a person where an accident at work or an industrial disease was contracted before 5 July 1948.

There are several sources of information and advice about benefits. They include Age Concern, local DSS offices, Citizens' Advice Bureaux, various local, voluntary, welfare-advice centres, DSS leaflets, post offices and libraries. Despite the wide range of help available there are still difficulties. Sometimes access to advice centres is not easy because of their location. There has tended to be too many leaflets, although these have been recently revised with improvements. Telephone directories might help by entering the centres under general headings such as 'Welfare Benefits' or 'Advice'. There is a free national telephone service 'Freeline Social Security', which gives advice on all aspects of the DSS benefit scheme. The Freephone number is 0800 666 555.

REFERENCES

Abrams, M. (1983) Changes in the lifestyles of the elderly 1959–1982. *Social Trends*, **14**, 11–16.
Fiegehen, G.C. (1986) Income after retirement. *Social Trends* **16**, 13–18.
HMSO (1987) *Social Trends* No 17.

6 Dynamics of
health and ageing

Natural ageing is a subtle and little understood process. There is no point in time when a particular person becomes old and yet the differences between a 40-year-old and an 80-year-old are quite clear. Little is known about the mechanism of ageing but it is clearly important to get some understanding of the process and especially its relationship to disease. Aspects of ageing include not only physical and mental changes, but also social interactions.

NORMAL AGEING

Old age and the wish to prolong life have long had a fascination. The psalmist talked about a natural life length of three-score years and ten, and ever since people have desired to prolong this period. An increase in life expectancy has already occurred and the seventy-year-old point is being reached by many more people. Whether there has been an increase in life span – namely the total possible time that an individual can live – is, however, debatable. This may not be achievable and the next realistic aim must be to gain an increase in health expectancy so that full function is maintained for as long as possible.

The natural ageing process has been termed senescence and shows itself as Comfort (1964) points out as 'an increasing probability of death with chronological age'. This implies that changes take place in the body as time goes by in the absence of recognized disease. Very often, however, the process of senescence may also be accompanied by disease and one may well affect the other. Herein lies the problem. It is still unclear what is the nature of the effect that these two processes have on each other and indeed, whether there do in fact exist two quite separate ageing processes, one normal and the other abnormal.

Direct observation of the way in which people 'age' gives some clues. It is sometimes noted that an old person just 'fades away' and although disease is the likely reason it does hint that natural ageing is also at work. The time scale of ageing is also variable, and it is well known that people can appear much older than their chronological age would suggest, and similarly, many old people act and look much younger than their years. There is, therefore, often a difference between biological age and chronological age and in a person's life, this may alter as time progresses. This is of course not based on external appearance but on internal environment. It is also true that various organs age at different rates. People of the same age group are often compared to determine features of actual ageing, but this cross-sectional approach only confirms the variability of physiological responses to the passage of time and different lifestyles. Longitudinal studies of cohorts may reveal more information about how vitality is lost. Comfort (1964) makes the point that if we kept the vitality throughout life that we had at the age of twelve, about half of us would still be here in seven hundred years. We should be dying off like radioactive atoms at a random rate and we would have no specific age beyond which we know we were unlikely to live.

Many theories of ageing have been proposed to explain the process of natural senescence. No really convincing explanation has yet arrived, which is hardly surprising considering the complexity of the subject and the difficulties of experimentation. Some theories are, however, intriguing. Hippocrates thought that old age was due to loss of body heat. The anatomist Theodore Swann considered that a vital life material was gradually lost and this contributed to ageing. Observations that social class can affect longevity supported a view that environment can affect the rate of ageing. In experimental animals it has been shown that exposure to radiation and overfeeding can both lead to premature death (McCay, 1952). Genetic influences can affect the likelihood of attaining extreme old age as the study of certain family pedigrees shows. The Trevellyan family, for instance, constantly reach great ages. Different species have different life spans, for example, elephants live longer than mice. Is this because of different rates of cell division or an inherently slower rate of ageing or both? The idea of lethal genes which evolutionarily slipped through the net of natural selection because they were late acting and so beyond the normal reproducing period, was advanced by Medawar (1952). These have been taken further by Kirkwood (1988) and are certainly ingenious.

These theories, based to some extent on observation, do not, however, deepen understanding of the process. Neither do other theories based more on conjecture. For instance, the 'programme theory' where senescence is regarded as an inevitable stage in the sequence that begins with fertilization and carries on through foetal life, birth, childhood, youth and on to maturity, is again unlikely, because the relatively small variation in the age at which developing organisms attain each specific stage in development contrasts with the wide variations in the age of onset of many of the features of old age. For instance, the appearance of an occasional grey hair before normal growth is finished is hardly consistent with the programme theory. The consistent age of onset of the menopause on the other hand is supportive evidence. Furthermore, the toxic theory that argues that poisonous substances accumulate in the organism and produce dysfunction and death, fails to account for the anatomical specificity of many age-dependent changes. The wear-and-tear theory likens old age to machine failure, but it is impossible to apply this idea to such conditions as greying of hair and arcus senilis.

The theories described so far are basically non-biological. In an attempt to introduce biological principles, interest has centred on so-called error theories and there are several of these. Evidence is seen of ageing in various microscopic elements in the body. Extracellular connective tissue may show changes in structure and cells themselves may become defective. On a widespread scale, as with the loss or greying of hair, numerous cells develop defects more-or-less simultaneously. Burch (1974) considers that many of these macroscopic manifestations of ageing reflect a relational disturbance: that is, errors of synthesis of recognition proteins occur in one or sometimes several central, growth-control cells and the mutant products of their descendent cells attack target cells that bear complementary recognition proteins. The macrocytic consequences of the attack are observed in the target cells, which in some instances are distributed at many anatomical sites. This points to a controlling central factor, the hypothalamus. Two rather similar theories have been proposed along these lines: the autoimmune and the autoaggressive theories. Both theories are complex, but basically the idea of the autoimmune theory is that mutations occur that produce immunological intolerance resulting in self-impairment of cells and, in certain situations, death. The autoaggressive theory is more fundamental and postulates mutation, not in the system that controls the normal immune response to particular antigens, but in the system that normally controls the size and growth of target tissues throughout the body.

These ideas are intriguing and obviously open up the way to more fundamental research. It is still difficult, however, to see a clear distinction between normal ageing or senescence and that associated with disease. Possibly ageing consists in the main of a constellation of specific age-dependent, autoaggressive disorders that encompass both physiological and pathological ageing. The reader is referred to an excellent discussion of the subject by Professor J. Grimley Evans (Evans, 1988).

Despite these conjectures, in recent years considerable attention has focused on the modification of those aspects of ageing previously thought to be normal and unalterable (Rowe and Kahn, 1987). This has proved to have very practical implications. When considering age-related losses in both mental and physical capacity, the substantial heterogenicity of older persons has sometimes been forgotten. Although wide variation of some biological parameters is a mark of senescence, there is evidence that the role of age in such losses has often been overstated and that a major component of many so-called age-associated reductions can be explained in terms of life style, habit, diet and an array of psycho-social variables. The concept of 'normal' ageing arose when considering evidence of the effects of age on such clinically relevant entities as hearing, vision, renal function, glucose tolerance, systolic blood pressure, bone density and immune function. It appeared that there were inevitable changes present that were time-related although not necessarily due to time. This idea of normal ageing can lead to negativism as it gives the impression that the decline is inevitable, and indeed harmless, and so inhibits attempts at its modification. To counteract this, it is necessary to distinguish between usual ageing and successful ageing. This allows a more positive approach and by studying successful ageing the factors involved in this can then be elucidated. There is evidence, for instance, that suggests that much of the observed carbohydrate intolerance in older people may be caused by factors other than biological ageing, and that modification to diet and exercise may substantially reduce the rate of these changes. Similarly, it is possible to modify the development of osteoporosis with age by, for instance, instituting moderate exercise programmes. Where mental impairment is present, attention and motivation may improve with appropriate intervention. Psychological factors are also relevant and autonomy is important to the wellbeing of an old person. The extent to which such autonomy is encouraged or denied may be a major determinant in whether ageing is usual or successful. Social support is also necessary in successful ageing and may work by mitigating some of the ill effects of changing circumstances sometimes seen in later life.

These ideas linking usual ageing, successful ageing and the effects of disease when considering the natural history of old age are important and have care implications. The possibility of modifying the process of ageing by such vehicles as diet, exercise, life style, social support and maintenance of personal autonomy need to be accepted as part of a philosophy of health promotion in old age.

CHANGES IN SPECIFIC SYSTEMS IN OLD AGE

The effects of usual ageing sometimes merge with the abnormal and it is important to recognize what is controllable and what is uncontrollable. Some physical changes are obvious. Height is reduced and the body becomes smaller due to loss of body mass. Very often there is thoracic kyphosis, particularly in women. The hair becomes grey and in both men and women may be lost. Muscle power for sustained effort is reduced and the grip may become poor. Teeth are lost, or at least the gums retract, giving the so-called long-in-the-tooth appearance. Control of body temperature is harder to achieve and old people easily become cold. Patterns of sleep alter and night cramps occur with greater frequency. The voice changes and may grow thin due to loss of elasticity of the laryngeal cartilage and muscle. A full account of changes associated with ageing is given in textbooks of geriatric medicine. Some practical points are, however, given here.

Nervous system
There is a decline in neurological function with increasing age. Tendon and superficial reflexes are sometimes absent in old people, particularly ankle jerks. Anderson (1971) found abdominal reflexes absent in about 20% of men and over 50% of women in the Rutherglen series. Sensory perception may be reduced in old age, particularly in the lower extremities. The normal pattern is for reduced sensory discrimination, particularly in the ability to perceive changes in temperature. The decreased sensory perception that occurs is not necessarily neurological in origin. Light touch, for example, can be affected by the presence of oedema, which may make sensory testing extremely difficult. Though vibration sense is commonly lost in the lower extremities it is rather unusual for it to be accompanied by a loss of position sense, if the latter is tested for properly. Obviously patient compliance influences the testing for position sense to a large degree. Most clinicians would regard true loss of position sense as being pathological. Indeed, it must never be accepted that changes are necessarily due to ageing alone and consideration must be given to the possibility of there being disease present. The brain shows some cell loss, but less than previously assumed, and not all types of brain cell are affected. There are also changes in neurotransmitter systems. Changes in the dendrites may be more significant than in the cells.

Special senses
Herbst and Humphrey (1981), using pure-tone audiometry, assessed the prevalence of hearing impairment in a sample of elderly people aged 70 or more, living at home. They found that 60% of the sample were deaf. This is higher than previously assumed. Undoubtedly there has been a serious underestimate of the level. There are, of course, possible pathological causes, and these are discussed in Chapter 19.

Eyesight deteriorates as age advances and becomes symptomatic by the mid-forties. Drooping of the upper lids is common in elderly people. The lens becomes increasingly opaque and less elastic, which results in decreased accommodation range and final loss of accommodation power by the age of 65 to 70. The pupillary reflexes become slower and the diameter of the pupil decreases. Recovery from glare takes longer and there is a deterioration in dark adaptation and colour vision.

Digestive system
Deterioration of the digestive system is not particularly marked in old age. Diseases of the liver and biliary tract are, however, generally regarded

as becoming more common with increasing age. Gastrointestinal disturbances may be increased and there is a tendency towards constipation.

Respiratory system
Respiratory efficiency is reduced along with the total lung volume.
Oxygen diffusion in the lungs may be impaired and tissue utilization is
less efficient. The respiratory reserve capacity is reduced, probably partly
due to impaired movement of the thoracic cage.

Cardiovascular system
Systemic arterial blood pressure does not necessarily rise with age.
Williams (1973) recorded the blood pressures of 270 unselected patients
over 75 years of age (86 men and 184 women). The means of the readings
in the various age groups are shown in Table 6.1. These findings indicate
that levels do not increase even amongst the very old, although the wide
standard deviation may mean that the picture is complicated. There was
little difference between the sexes. Survival seems to be more likely if the
blood pressure is not high or too low. These people probably represent a
special group in the population where blood pressure was stable.

One of the problems, however, with looking at the relationship between arterial pressure and age is that most of the studies, like the one
quoted, are cross-sectional and not longitudinal. It may well be that many
of the patients in whom high blood pressure has produced end-organ
damage will have already died by the time they reach 75 so the group

Table 6.1 Mean level of blood pressure (with standard deviations) for men and
women over 75 years old

Age group	Mean systolic and standard deviation in mm of mercury	Mean diastolic and standard deviation in mm of mercury
(a) Male		
75–79	155 ± 24.77	86 ± 10.9
80–84	162 ± 24.80	87 ± 11.53
85–89	171 ± 31.37	90 ± 12.14
90+	142 ± 26.39	81 ± 14.72
All ages 75+	159 ± 26.25	86 ± 11.28
(b) Female		
75–79	163 ± 23.64	91 ± 8.84
80–84	158 ± 23.24	90 ± 13.63
85–89	159 ± 25.34	90 ± 12.65
90+	156 ± 11.40	88 ± 4.47
All ages 75+	160 ± 23.57	90 ± 11.48

Sample: 270 cases (86 men; 184 women)

Source: Williams (1973)

reported above represents survivors. It is possible that in the over-80s high blood pressure is in fact associated with increased survival and the significance of high blood pressure in this group may need reconsidering.

The arteries in old age become thickened and hard, probably due to an increase in arterial collagen, and the collagen that is laid down is less elastic due to more molecular cross-linking. This results in the arteries themselves being less compliant. Veins are less affected by ageing. Thoracic kyphosis often displaces the apex beat of the heart and this may also mask emphysema. As many as two-thirds of patients aged over 70 have systolic-ejection murmurs over the aortic area.

Haemoglobin
Williams *et al.* (1972) estimated haemoglobin levels in 286 patients over 75 years of age. A histogram of the distribution is shown in Fig. 6.1. The differences in haemoglobin levels between the sexes in ages up to 75 years has frequently been commented upon. From the study quoted, it would appear that this influence extends well beyond this age.

Endocrine system
It is difficult to assess the precise effects of ageing on the various endocrine glands. This is partly due to the fact that routine measurement of endocrine function in elderly people is done at one point in time and dynamic tests of function are rarely carried out. Thyroid function is thought to decrease with age, but there is no clear evidence for this. There is some evidence that the stress response in the pituitary–adrenal axis is diminished in elderly people, though under non-stress conditions cortisone measurements are normal. Secretion of sex hormones declines with age and this affects secondary sex features, such as the breasts, which tend to atrophy. There is a very comprehensive review of current thinking on the endocrine system in old age by Green in Pathy's Textbook on Geriatric Medicine (Pathy, 1985).

Renal system
Changes do occur in renal function. There is evidence of a decline in glomerular filtration and renal blood flow. The acid/base balance is hard to maintain in old age.

The skin
Changes in the skin are very noticeable. Environmental factors can affect these changes and prolonged exposure to sunlight can accelerate the process. Skin ageing also varies from person to person, and it is possible that some hereditary influence is at work. The changes consist mainly of atrophy of the epidermis with an increase in pigmentation and degenerative changes in the collagenous and elastic fibres of the dermis.

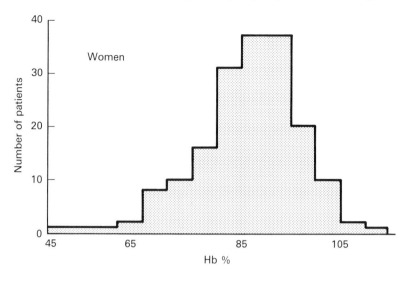

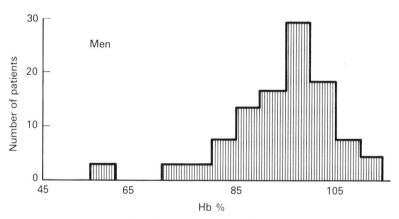

Haemoglobin values (100% = 14.8 g/100 ml) in the study;
popluation aged 75 and over.

Figure 6.1 Haemoglobin values (Williams *et al.*, 1972)

Pigmented areas are seen more frequently and there is a high incidence of small papillomata. The skin looks thinner, shows more wrinkles and appears lax and dry. The subcutaneous fat may be reduced and the skin sometimes has a loose, hanging appearance. The nails grow at a slower rate and may be more brittle. There may be a reduction in sweat due to atrophy of the sweat glands. Hair follicles are reduced in density and the hair is markedly thinner, but curiously rarely completely absent. Greying of the hair due to loss of melanin pigment is almost universal and the process can start at an early age.

PSYCHOLOGICAL ASPECTS OF AGEING

As well as physical changes, old age brings with it an alteration in psychological outlook. This is variable, but certain characteristics are recognizable and these probably arise from the cumulative effects of psychological adaption in earlier stages of life. The pathway from early adulthood through middle adulthood to the pre-retirement phase of 60 to 65 usually consists of a complex series of events that contribute to psychological ageing. Sex differences are apparent in the process, but probably less so now when increasing numbers of women have careers. Women do, however, tend to live longer than men, and the psycho-social transition can be different. Both men and women have to adjust to the eventual departure of children to live their own independent lives. Retirement needs coping with and for women especially, there is the prospect of widowhood. Social-class differences are also present. Manual workers reach the summit of their working lives early, whereas professional workers do not reach their maximum working capacity until much later. Successful psychological reassessment in middle age can have a bearing on attitudes in old age. Realization that some ambitions will not be fulfilled and the adoption of realistic aims for the remaining time available are important in middle age and lead to a more contented old age. Many adjustments are necessary. Some men despair of their physical decline in middle age, whereas others are proud of their relative youth. Women, too, become more aware of their husband's health and think of the possibilities of his dying. They rehearse for widowhood, and sometimes plan along these lines. For instance, they may want to move into a smaller, more convenient house and look to their own financial security. These may of course be merely sensible arrangements taken in response to changing circumstances. Hopefully, adjustments will be made to these problems before the major hurdle of retirement is reached. There is a risk at this time that disengagement might occur and newly retired people might withdraw from the mainstream of life. Ideally this should not happen and old people should maintain their interest and activity, certainly in what has come to be known as 'young old age' from 65 to 75. Eventually, however, a stage is sometimes reached when an old person cannot cope with the demands of everyday living and becomes dependent on others. Some adapt to this, whereas others resent the whole concept of ageing and fear having to rely on others for help. In some cases, role reversal takes place with the elderly individual's children adopting the parental role, the elderly person being placed in the dependent-child relationship. This often causes problems for the children as well as for the elderly individual. People living by themselves, particularly if their personality was originally introverted, gradually withdraw from social contact and become isolated. When depression is present or physical neglect occurs, these people can become quite desolate and may cut themselves off from help. Intelligence itself does not show much decline with ageing but the capacity to solve new problems deteriorates. Faced with the fear that they may no longer be able to solve problems, some old people may tend to become apathetic and often do not seek help even when this is readily available. Nevertheless there are many positive psychological features of ageing, especially today. The provision of good pension and security have allowed many to use this freedom to enable late development and the opportunity to fulfill ambitions previously denied by the demands of a working life.

CHANGING CHARACTERISTICS OF ILLNESS IN OLD AGE

Probably the first thing to say about any illness in old age is that it needs to be looked at in physical, mental and social terms. The interdependence between the patient's environment, and his or her mental and physical state is often crucially important. Illness may often be due to a combination of problems and management must take into account all these factors. Pathology, of course, is more common in old age and there is a general increase in morbidity. Some diseases are age-related. Generalized arteriosclerosis and osteoporosis are two examples. Not surprisingly, multiple disability is so common as to be almost the rule. Thomas (1968), in running a clinic for elderly people, found that more than 80% of his group had multiple disability and numerous other surveys have supported this finding. Many of the conditions found are degenerative in type but some are amenable to treatment. Many are minor, but the problem is that the presence of several of these can set up a vicious circle, resulting in a reduction in a patient's functional capacity, and severe disablement ensues. An example of conditions interacting in this way is obesity affecting osteoarthritic knees and possible cardiac impairment. The presence of anaemia may also affect adversely the course of many conditions.

Multiple symptomatology is also a common finding. Elderly patients the dependent-child relationship. This often causes problems for the questioning. Some symptoms impair health more than others. In the author's survey of over-75-year-olds, dizziness or giddiness was a common symptom occurring more frequently in patients of poor effective health. Forgetfulness is another distressing symptom of old age. Symptoms must also be interpreted differently in old age. Ferguson Anderson (1967), for instance, attaches the same significance to confusion in an old person as to convulsions in a baby, that is, it might be produced by a number of causes, including anything that increases the temperature. Old people may have a different threshold of pain and may complain of it less frequently. They also do not seem to appreciate thirst as acutely. Temperature changes may also not be noticed. Physical signs of illness in the aged need assessing differently. The changes already described which occur with natural ageing, influence, for instance, the measurement of heart size and position.

Illnesses in old age may have unusual clinical presentations. Infections often progress insidiously and may only be discovered at an advanced stage. In some infections the temperature does not necessarily always rise and the white-cell count remains normal. Tuberculosis sometimes presents as no more than general weakness and tiredness. Non-specific failure to thrive can be due to bacteraemia. Presentation of both thyroid over- and underactivity may be very atypical in old age.

Heart disease, too, has various presentations. Angina is relatively uncommon; myocardial infarction occurs but is difficult to diagnose clinically as pain only occurs in about a quarter of the cases and the attack may be asymptomatic. Confusion and restlessness are usually present in acute infarction and most forms of heart failure. Diabetes mellitus can also present atypically and may first be noticed as bed-wetting or incontinence. An illness in old age can be complicated by such factors as hypothermia, sensitivity to drugs and subnutrition. Dehydration easily occurs and can cloud the clinical picture.

UNREPORTED NEED

Old age also brings with it some changes in attitude and behaviour. An important example is the phenomenon of unreported need. This was first described by Williamson *et al.* in 1964. Many studies have subsequently confirmed these findings (Williams *et al.* 1972; Currie *et al.*, 1974; Freedman, Charlewood and Dodds 1978; Vetter, Jones and Victor, 1984). It would seem that old people cannot tell when they are unwell and in need of help. This means that disease is not detected at an early stage and, as Ferguson Anderson (1967) puts it, 'there is an iceberg of unreported illness amongst the old people in the community'. Why should this be so? Several reasons have been advanced. There is a general apathy and lack of initiative in old people and they have the idea that such conditions as breathlessness and ankle swelling are not due to illness but are an integral part of old age. Old people may find it difficult to attend the doctor's surgery because of lack of transport or inconvenient hours; but perhaps it is more a fear of what might happen when they arrive and many have an aversion to being admitted to hospital or undergoing investigation. Again, they may feel that they do not want to trouble the doctor with conditions they think are basically untreatable. It seems a problem primarily of urban society and it is interesting to contemplate why this should be. Perhaps isolation is more common in towns than in the country.

What are the sorts of disability that are unreported and unknown to the doctor? Although in all surveys serious conditions such as malignant disease, heart failure and diabetes were found, many of the problems were relatively minor. These would include such conditions as hallux valgus, toenail deformity, varicose veins, skin lesions, inguinal hernia, osteoarthritis and Dupuytren's contracture. In women various conditions of the genitourinary system, like vulvovaginitis, cervical polyp, prolapse, urethral caruncle and urinary infections were found. Perhaps this is due to the intimate nature of the symptoms and old ladies' reluctance to discuss such 'private problems'. In men, hydrocele and prostatic symptoms were often unreported for the same reason. Eye and ear conditions also figure largely in the findings, including deafness caused by the infinitely treatable wax in the ear. Many mental conditions, too, tend to be unreported.

REFERENCES

Anderson, W.F. (1971) *Practical Management of the Elderly*, Blackwell Scientific Publications, Oxford and Edinburgh.

Burch, P.J.R. (1974) The biological nature of ageing. *Symposia of Geriatric Medicine*, **3**, West Midlands Institute of Geriatric Medicine and Gerontology.

Comfort, A. (1964) *Ageing. The Biology of Senescence*, Routledge and Kegan Paul, London.

Currie, G., MacNeill, R.M., Walker, J.G., Barnie, E. and Mudie, E.W. (1974) Medical and social screening of patients aged 70 to 72 by an urban general practice health team, *Br. Med. J.*, **2**, 108–11.

Evans, J.G. (1988) Ageing and disease. In *Research and the Ageing Population*. Evered, D. and Whelan, J. (Eds), Wiley, Chichester.

Ferguson Anderson, W. (1967) *Practical Management of the Elderly*, Blackwell Scientific Publications, Oxford and Edinburgh.

Freedman, G.R., Charlewood, J.E. and Dodds, P.A. (1978) Screening the aged in general practice. *J. R. Coll. Gen. Pract.*, **24**, 421–5.

Herbst, K.G. and Humphrey, C. (1981) Prevalence of hearing impairment in the elderly living at home. *J. R. Coll. Gen. Pract.*, **31**, 155–60.

Kirkwood, T.B.L. (1988) The nature and causes of ageing. In *Research and the Ageing Population*. Evered, D. and Whelan, J. (Eds), Wiley, Chichester.

McCay, C.M. (1952) In *Problems of Ageing*. Lansing, A.I. (Ed.) Williams and Wilkins, Baltimore.

Medawar, P.B. (1952) *An Unsolved Problem of Biology*. H.K. Lewis, London.

Pathy, M.S.J. (1985) *Principles and Practice of Geriatric Medicine*, John Wiley and Sons, Chichester.

Rowe, J.W. and Kahn, R.L. (1987) Human ageing. Usual and successful. *Science*, **237**, 143–9.

Thomas, P. (1968) Experience of two preventative clinics for the elderly. *Br. Med.*

J., **2**, 357–60.

Vetter, N.J., Jones, D.E. and Victor, C.R. (1984) Affect of health visitors working with elderly patients in general practice: a randomised controlled trial. *Br. Med. J.*, **288**, 369–72.

Williams, E.I. (1973) A socio-medical study of patients over 75 years in an urban general practice. Unpublished MD thesis, Manchester University.

Williams, E.I., Bennett, F.M., Nixon, J.V. *et al.* (1972) Socio-medical study of patients over 75 in general practice. *Br. Med. J.*, **2**, 445–8.

Williamson, J., Stokoe, I.H., Gray, S. *et al.* (1964) Old people at home: their unreported needs. *Lancet*, **i**, 1117–20.

7 Social vulnerability

SOCIAL INDEPENDENCE

Everyone needs the basic requirements for day-to-day living. These include shelter, food, clothes, warmth, toilet facilities, cleanliness and safety. There is also the necessity for privacy, which old people in particular find very important, and the ability to express emotional warmth, and some status at least in one's family or neighbourhood. Most also require a range of interests to be able to gain personal satisfaction and enjoyment. This means being able to undertake certain personal and domestic tasks (Table 7.1 and 7.2), together with having the physical ability to perform social activities. Happily all of these are usually present in later life and enable most old people to live independently in the community. When old people themselves are unable to undertake these activities, relatives, friends and neighbours are usually able to supply the help needed. As a result most live contentedly in the community in a state of equilibrium, although this is sometimes only maintained with difficulty and personal cost to carers and supporters.

WHAT GOES WRONG?

Two types of situation can arise that cause a change in this social equilibrium. Both can produce domestic deterioration – one insidiously and the other dramatically. The first is where, although basic care is still being given, a time arrives when personal and domestic tasks become too demanding for the old person to undertake and there then develops a slow but steady lowering in the quality of living, although this may not be immediately appreciated. The second is when a crisis occurs due to a sudden breakdown in the provision of basic care.

Isaacs and Neville (1972), in their study of the Scottish Health Services, detail in their book, *The Measurement of Need in Old People*, three categories of vulnerable old person. The first is the protected category, in which the old person is in an institution and therefore protected from social problems. The second is the defended category, in which the old person is cared for by a relative and is thus in a state of social equilibrium and defended from the problems associated with care. The third is the defeated category and this is where an old person fails to receive any sort of care or where relatives suffer an intolerable strain in providing it.

The ideas of the defended and the defeated are important because with a defensible situation, help can be given to maintain the old person in the community, usually by providing short-interval or critical-interval care; however, the defeated position usually requires admission to a protected environment, either in a hospital or welfare home. Isaacs and Neville (1972) found that for every severely disabled old person in hospital there were two at home who had a similar degree of disability and therefore were on the brink of changing from being defended to being defeated. This meant that care was still being given, but presumably at great cost to the provider.

It is with the defeated situation that the doctor or social worker is usually involved, but the process of change from the defended equilibrium to the defeated or near-defeated position is often gradual and recognition of this process is important because it allows help to be provided and breakdown avoided. The actual defeat is usually a crisis that requires immediate and urgent help. These two situations will be discussed separately although they are usually part of the same process.

Gradual deterioration in social equilibrium

Examples of personal and domestic tasks essential to normal daily living are listed in Tables 7.1 and 7.2. Although inability to undertake any of

Table 7.1 Examples of self care

1. Cutting toenails	7. Getting in and out of bed
2. Climbing stairs	8. Getting to lavatory
3. Using public transport	9. Shaving/combing hair
4. Bathing	10. Washing
5. Getting out of doors	11. Feeding yourself
6. Getting around house	

Source: Barlow and Matthews (1978)

Table 7.2 Examples of domestic tasks

1. Decorating	8. Sewing
2. Carrying out minor repairs	9. Washing clothes
3. Cleaning windows outside	10. Sweeping floors
4. Climbing stairs	11. Unscrewing jars
5. Washing the paintwork	12. Cooking
6. Cleaning windows inside	13. Using frying pan
7. Washing floors	14. Making a cup of tea

Source: Barlow and Matthews (1978)

these can produce hardship, failure to be able to perform such important functions as washing, feeding and toileting are the most serious. Where there is difficulty with one task it is likely that there is similar difficulty with another that involves the same type of movement. Indeed, certain tasks can be grouped together so that when one of the tasks cannot be performed it is probable that the others cannot be performed either. For instance, this would apply to particular personal tasks associated with mobility in the home such as climbing stairs, moving around the house, getting in and out of bed and going to the lavatory. Similarly, there is a second group that includes those tasks involving the ability to flex the spine. Examples would be getting in and out of a bath, cutting toenails and getting on and off a bus. Finally, a group can involve tasks associated with moving the hands, such as shaving, washing and feeding. So it is likely that a person who experiences difficulty with one task also experiences difficulty with others in the same group. The recognition of these associations may be important when assessing functional ability.

Similar groups can also be formed for domestic tasks, although this is complicated by sex roles. For example, it is traditional for women to be associated with cooking and washing and men to be associated with doing repairs. Even so, broad divisions can be made between light and heavy housework. It is often important to recognize that if an old person is finding difficulty in one task, he or she may also be finding difficulty with others of a similar nature. The full extent of the deterioration may be unperceived unless this is recognized.

Many of these problems may be minor at first, and decline usually starts with activities outside the home. There are numerous examples. It may become impossible to continue taking the dog for a walk, or the garden is too difficult to manage and hence mowing the lawn and weeding are neglected. Slowly household maintenance also suffers, and eventually simple cleaning is overlooked. Long-distance mobility becomes impossible. A visit may be made to the local shops, but longer journeys to buy special items are avoided; hobbies and visits to clubs stop. Help for this type of problem is usually provided by neighbours and relatives, but if no-one is available, standards begin to fall.

Some problems are more subtle and hence more difficult for a family to solve. It may not be easy to perceive that old people are failing to keep up with changing economic circumstances and are not assimilating new information. Thus pension rates change, licensing fees for television are raised and these facts need to be understood. Poverty has long been a problem of old age and this may not only be due to lack of money, but also to having expenditure ridiculously out of proportion to necessity. The house may be too large and a burden to maintain. Some old people have financial commitments to relatives that are obviously unfair and cause a considerable amount of stress and worry. On the other hand, many come from a thrifty generation who have always been taught to save for a rainy day. In extreme old age, they still feel they need to save or at least not spend 'extravagantly', even though it seems obvious to other people that this frugality is quite unnecessary. They are reluctant to buy clothes and fuel for heat even though they have adequate resources to do this. Savings preclude help from the State and it is sometimes hard for relatives to persuade an old person to spend more of the reserve money on the basic necessities of life.

Retirement may bring problems. A man's adjustment to being constantly round the house and his wife's acceptance of it are not easily achieved. Quarrels may ensue and result in rifts within a family with long-lasting repercussions on the standard of care being given. Family disputes can take other forms and it is well known that as age advances some old people can become extremely unreasonable. Difficult character traits that were perhaps accepted in earlier years can become exaggerated to such an extent that an old person can become awkward and vindictive. Particular likes and dislikes can be taken to relatives and neighbours. Sometimes an elderly person may be in a position to make life extremely difficult for these people. The result is a lack of sympathy and the old person fails to receive the necessary help.

Minor mental deterioration may not be recognized and subtle behavioural changes may pass unnoticed until they become a serious problem. A good example of this is a tendency to hoard. In the early stages this may amount to nothing more than an exaggeration of a natural instinct to gather supplies of food, or an old man's eccentric hobby of collecting newspapers or periodicals, but once the house becomes a fantastic jumble of irrelevant items, things have gone too far and the situation is abnormal.

Sexual problems sometimes arise and an old man may become very demanding of his now unsympathetic wife. His attentions are perhaps turned on other women in the immediate circle and although this is often regarded as playfulness and treated as a joke, it can be embarrassing and unwelcome. Although the family tends to cover up the real nature of the problem in these circumstances, a reassuring and positive response by health and social workers to a call for help is very necessary.

The phenomenon of the captive spouse is also seen. As time goes on, one member of the marital pair is likely to become ill and in need of care. This involves the other partner in a considerable additional burden. Not only are there the normal household **duties**, but also the extra commitments of caring physically for a sick partner. This creates the situation where the well partner has to withdraw from all previous outside activities and care becomes a full-time occupation. There are times in late old age when a man or woman may be working harder than at any other time in earlier life, and although the situation may appear to an outsider to be very well managed it must be realized that this is happening at great cost.

Social as well as physical help is often desperately needed. Particularly tragic is the plight of aged parents with a physically or mentally handicapped son or daughter living with them. The offspring is often ageing as well and needing more and not less help.

Outside influences can affect the standard of life of old people. For instance, long waiting lists in the National Health Service can have more damaging effects on the aged than on other sections of the community. In Britain today there is a multiracial society. At present the proportion of old people is not high amongst some of the ethnic groups, but this is gradually changing. Little is known about such things as unreported need, social isolation and carer responses to stress among these members of society.

These are examples of social problems that are often part of a gradual decline. The process is slow. It may take years before it is realized how far standards have fallen. As with illness, many such problems are unreported and often multiple. Some are quite intractable and these have to be accepted. Trigger difficulties of relatively minor degree can sometimes plunge the situation into crisis, and it is necessary to watch out for these. Tension between an old person and a carer, for instance, can mean withdrawal of care. In the three-generation household, where overcrowding exists and there is no privacy for children, problems at school can develop. If this occurs resentment can arise between a grandparent and daughter-in-law, which may lead to care problems.

Acute social crises

Acute social crises occur when there is breakdown in the provision of basic care and action is then usually necessary by the caring services. The nature of the crisis usually depends on the underlying causes. These can be broadly divided into problems with the old person, problems with helpers, problems with the environment and failures in communication. There is considerable overlap between these factors, but for convenience they will be examined separately.

Patient or client problems

An old person may be living alone or with relatives. Where help is available, difficulties occur when the level of care required increases to such a point that it is impossible for the helpers to cope any more. Where an old person lives alone without help it is when he/she can no longer manage that the trouble occurs. In these situations where the problem is fundamentally patient- or client-centred, it is usually illness that precipitates the breakdown. This can be physical or mental and may be either major or minor, and it often does not matter which. The important point is that as a result of the illness, basic care can no longer be provided. Minor episodes of influenza or gastroenteritis can have the same effect as heart failure or acute bronchitis. Usually major illness such as stroke demands admission to hospital and this temporarily eases the situation, but hardship can arise when the patient is discharged home. However, sometimes even minor illness can result in the patient being admitted to hospital as social care is not possible at home. Progressive illnesses such as chronic nerve degeneration involve slow deterioration and crisis then occurs less obviously, but even so a point is reached where more care is needed than it is possible to provide. Terminal illness may also produce similar urgent problems. Falls and accidents may bring sudden social incapacity. An old lady may be managing very well until a slip on the ice results in a fractured wrist. Treatment at a casualty department is easy but the patient is quite unable to cope when she arrives back home. Sometimes admission to a welfare home is required, though often only for a short time. Other injuries, such as a fractured femur, demand a longer period of rehabilitation. Mental illnesses frequently cause social problems. It is not uncommon for old people to attempt suicide and this may be a symptom of their inability to cope with the demands of self-care. Behavioural problems such as increasing antagonism towards neighbours may also present as acute social crises. Failing vision and deafness may render patients incapable of looking after themselves, especially when the handling of drugs and self-administration of treatment are needed. All the situations discussed in the section on non-crisis situations ('Gradual deterioration in social equilibrium') pp. 56–9 may flare up into acute crises. Particularly vulnerable are patients who are housefast.

Helper problems

Patient difficulties can have an effect on the health and level of tolerance of helpers. Admission of old people to hospital is sometimes due to friends and relatives being unable to cope any further. Sanford (1975) found this to be so in 12% of all geriatric admissions to University College Hospital, London and the Whittingham Hospital. The person principally involved with home support was interviewed in 50 such cases. The causes of inability to cope were identified and the supporters were asked to assess which of these would have to be alleviated to restore a tolerable situation at home. Forty-six of the carers were able to do this. The problems identified were divided into three groups:

1. dependant's behaviour pattern
2. supporter's own limitations
3. environmental conditions

(See Tables 7.3, 7.4 and 7.5.)

Table 7.3 Analysis of Group 1 problems identified (dependants' behaviour patterns)

	Frequency (percentage of cases)	Tolerance (percentage of supporters able to tolerate problem)
Sleep disturbance	62	16
Night wandering	24	24
Micturition	24	17
Shouting	10	20
Incontinence of faeces	56	43
Incontinence of urine	54	81
Falls	58	52
Inability to get out of bed unaided	52	35
Inability to get into bed unaided	50	40
Inability to get on commode unaided	36	22
Inability to get off commode unaided	38	21
Dangerous, irresponsible behaviour	32	38
Inability to walk at all	16	13
Personality conflicts	26	54
Physically aggressive behaviour	18	44
Inability to dress unaided	44	77
Inability to wash and/or shave unaided	54	93
Inability to communicate	16	50
Daytime wandering	12	33
Inability to manage stairs unaided	10	60
Inability to feed unaided	12	67
Blindness	2	0

Source: Sanford (1975)

Table 7.4 Analysis of Group 2 problems identified (supporters' own limitations)

	Frequency (percentage of cases)	Tolerance (percentage of supporters able to tolerate problem)
Anxiety/depression	52	65
Personality conflicts	26	54
Insufficient strength for lifting	22	73
Rheumatoid/osteoarthritis	12	67
Back strain	8	100
Bronchitis	6	33
Embarrassment	4	0
Other	12	67

Source: Sanford (1975)

Table 7.5 Analysis of Group 3 problems identified (environmental and social conditions)

	Frequency (percentage of cases)	Tolerance (percentage of supporters able to tolerate problem)
Restriction of social life	42	57
Inability to leave dependant for more than one hour	28	71
Stairs within accommodation	26	85
Financial disadvantage	4	0
Other	4	0

Source: Sanford (1975)

Of the difficulties that carers felt unable to tolerate, 80% were in Group One, 11% were in Group Two and 9% were in Group Three. The degrees of tolerance varied for different types of situation. Sleep disturbance and faecal incontinence were, for instance, poorly tolerated in Group One as might be expected, but surprisingly urinary incontinence and inability to wash and dress were coped with reasonably well. It was clearly important that when patients are nursed at home a careful study has to be made of the factors most needing alleviation in the opinion of the helpers. Failure to recognize these can produce undue strain on families and although care may still be present, crises may be imminent and urgent action is often necessary to support these helpers.

An acute social emergency also arises when help ceases because of supporters' own limitations. This may be due to illness, either physical or mental in the helper, or when there are other commitments, such as nursing a sick child or dealing with other family matters. Sometimes the helper has to move away from the area due to a change in the spouse's occupation. Help may then stop altogether for the old person living alone. Even when a grandmother is living with a younger family, the arrival of a new baby may make it impossible, perhaps because of the shortage of space, for this to continue. The age of the helper may be important. Sometimes the supplier of basic care is elderly and may be unable to continue carrying the burden. In all situations, sometimes enough is enough, and particularly where a patient has mental illness the carers can come to the end of their tether and demand help.

Cases are found where basic care is insufficient despite family presence in the area. Isaacs and his co-authors in their book *Survival of the Unfittest* (1972) examine 39 examples of this type in some detail. The reasons why the social condition of old people was allowed to deteriorate despite the presence of available family were divided into four groups: preoccupation, dilemma, refusal and rejection.

Preoccupation

This was considered to be the reason why 17 of the 39 patients with children in the area failed to receive adequate care and is a circumstance that will be well understood by anyone having to deal with old people. The relatives provided as much care as they could and were anxious to give more, but were prevented from doing so by prior commitments from which they were quite unable to free themselves, or by an impediment that they could not overcome. These causes included health of the helper or care of another dependant.

Dilemma

This is where significant basic care is withheld because relatives, although capable and willing to give more help than they did, were forced to accept a different course in the interest of their own families. The dilemma of son and daughter in these circumstances is whether to give prior consideration to the needs of the parent or to those of their own family. Often an attempt was made to do both, but even so, the parent still received insufficient care. These situations are often full of anguish and feelings of guilt on the part of the offspring, and recrimination on the part of the old person. They are a rich source of family dispute and friction.

Refusal

This is where adequate care is absent because the old person is unwilling to receive it. In the series quoted by Isaacs *et al.*, they were almost all men and they were usually of an aggressive independent type, attracting very little love towards themselves and tending not to give any either. These patients would not admit that they needed help and did not like to put themselves in the situation of being obliged to anyone else. They were often in dreadful social circumstances and even when discovered by social workers were extremely difficult to help.

Rejection

This is where the patient seems to have been rejected by his or her children. This rejection was difficult to understand on first impression, but after further enquiry reasons were often found. Sometimes there was a family quarrel that went back for years and the rejection might initially have been on the parental side. Examples included a daughter thought not to have made a suitable marriage and a son who in the past had gone against parental wishes. Maybe the parents were ashamed of some event in the lives of their children as in the case of one son who had been to prison. Alcoholism in the parent or long-standing quarrels about money might drive children away. Second marriages sometimes caused problems. Initially, this might have seemed a good idea, but once one partner had become ill, the other one might feel aggrieved at having responsibilities of care after so short a time. Children may have disapproved of the second marriage and subsequently may have proved unwilling to share in the care of a stepmother or stepfather. First marriages never ran into this sort of difficulty.

Sometimes a problem in providing care for elderly people is that they do not like to be in another person's debt, even if these people are their own children. The presence of grandchildren is often good in overcoming these difficulties because of opportunities to reciprocate. If these are absent it might mean that the elderly couple become reluctant to ask for help and so a situation of neglect arises.

Environmental factors

These are usually associated with housing. There may be physical deterioration of a property and problems such as a leaking roof. Many old people live in houses that are in inner cities and these tend to become neglected. Vermin are attracted and may migrate to inhabited dwellings, particularly if these are dirty and poorly maintained. These areas are also happy hunting grounds for vandals, and inhabitants can be harrassed and disturbed. Eviction may happen when financial resources are low, and these threats to deprive someone of shelter can be extremely distressing. Old persons living with relatives may sometimes find themselves homeless when the family has to move to a smaller house with no spare room.

Co-operation problems

Crisis situations may occur when there is a failure of communication between the caring services. This may happen particularly when a hospital fails to inform the community social, medical and nursing services of an old person's discharge from hospital. This will be discussed in Chapter 15. Liaison should also be very close between hospital doctors and general practitioners. Lack of co-ordination between the domiciliary workers themselves may be a source of trouble. Clear demarcation of the role of a doctor and a social worker in a particular situation is sometimes not obvious and can only be overcome by person-to-person discussion about individual cases.

REFERENCES

Barlow, A. and Matthews, D. (1978) Need for the receipt of domiciliary social services amongst the elderly. Unpublished DHSS Statistical Paper, March.

Isaacs, B., Livingstone, M. and Neville, Y. (1972) *Survival of the Unfittest*, Routledge and Kegan Paul, London.

Isaacs, B. and Neville, Y. (1972) *The Measurement of Need in Old People*, Scottish Home and Health Department, Edinburgh.

Sanford, J.R.A. (1975) Tolerance of debility in elderly dependants by supporters at home: its significance for hospital practice. *Br. Med. J.*, **3**, 471–3.

8 Health-care provision

When considering the provision of services in the community, it is often helpful to consider real-life situations that have had to be helped by these services. Such a situation concerns a doctor who was called to see an old man late on a Friday afternoon. On arrival, the patient, in his late 70s, was found to be suffering from bronchitis and had been ill for some weeks. He lived alone in poor social circumstances. The doctor was received aggressively by relatives who had just called to see the patient: they were disturbed by the situation but because of other commitments, felt unable to give adequate care. Despite the fact that nobody had bothered to do anything about the old man's plight, they demanded that something be done, which in effect meant hospital admission. The problem was compounded by the fact that neither the doctor nor anyone from the primary health team had previous knowledge of the situation. The doctor's task was difficult: the bronchitis could have been treated at home if there had been someone to look after the patient; ideally social help and nursing help would be available but in this particular district and at this time, such care was not easily forthcoming. When contacted, the hospital was also difficult: no beds were available; the weekend lay ahead. The relatives were still reluctant to stay. Eventually the hospital did take the patient, but not without a great deal of persuasion and fairly universal frustration.

Anyone working in the community knows this type of situation and the story contains no exaggerations. How much better it would have been if the situation could have been prevented or foreseen and treatment and care initiated at an earlier stage! One of the principles of community care that this story also illustrates is the close links that exist between medical and social problems. Both are often present at the same time and it is usually merely a matter of degree whether the patient needs primarily medical (and this includes nursing) care or primarily social-services care (that is, provision of basic general care).

THE TRIANGLE OF CARE

When a person needs care there are three possible places where this can be given. These are in the patient's home, or in supervised accommo-

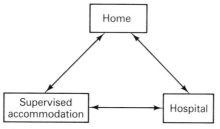

Figure 8.1 Triangle of care

dation, or in hospital. Supervised accommodation can be a local-authority welfare home, a private rest or nursing home, or sheltered housing. The place in which it is most appropriate for the patient to be really depends on the balance between the medical, nursing and social needs. It is of fundamental importance that these three places of care should be used appropriately. They form a triangle and there should be a freeflow of patients from one to the other (Fig. 8.1). Thus a patient may be admitted to hospital for acute care but may return to the community and his/her home via the half-way stage of a welfare home if social problems need resolving. Alternatively, patients may be discharged directly to their own homes with social and nursing care arranged. Several combinations of possibilities therefore exist. The hospital-at-home concept has proved to be an important experiment in this context.

DIFFICULTIES IN THE PROVISION OF CARE

Although the 'triangle of care' concept provides a neat framework in which to consider services for elderly people, in practice difficulties occur in all three areas and in what might be called the fourth side of the triangle, which is the need for workers to co-operate and communicate.

In primary care there are doctors who have little interest in elderly people and little training in geriatric care. Resettlement of patients discharged from hospital and their continuing care and rehabilitation are ignored. These deficiencies are reinforced by poor communication between GPs and domiciliary nursing services, as well as rehabilitation services in the community. The changes in the organization of general practice have sometimes militated against the interests of old people. Centralization of premises into health centres and the introduction of appointments systems have made it harder for an older person to consult. The change in attitude of doctors towards home visiting makes the sick old patient reluctant to call, although research shows that as many as half of the contacts between doctors and their senior patients occur at home. The increased use of repeat prescriptions sometimes means that elderly people miss out on continuing care and assessment.

Other difficulties arise because it is sometimes not possible to create suitable environmental arrangements for old people. Rehousing or adaptation of existing houses may not be possible. Transport may be hard to organize. Communication by telephone may be too expensive and public phone boxes vandalized. Social services such as home help and meals on wheels may be inadequate.

There may be too few trained workers available to deal with the complex variety of incidents presented by old people and there are also financial considerations that affect care provision. No criteria exist that lay down when an old person should be recommended for, and admitted to, welfare-home care. Leaving aside medical and social aspects, should economic grounds be the guiding factors? L.J. Opit, when writing in 1977, reported an investigation into the cost of domiciliary care by the home nursing service of 139 elderly sick patients. The data suggest that there may be little economic advantage in home care for elderly seriously disabled people. The revenue costs of care were equal to, or even greater than, the average hospital care of such patients. Opit took the highest domiciliary care costs and the lowest hospital costs. Nevertheless the point was made; there are clearly other factors to be taken into account but financial considerations will probably play an increasing part in influencing the provision of these services.

In the area of supervised accommodation, difficulties can also arise. In some localities the number of local-authority welfare homes is insufficient for the demand, although this has been eased in recent times by the increasing number of private rest homes available. Welfare homes are still, however, not being used appropriately and may be catering for old people who need a high degree of nursing care, or on the other hand, for people who could still be living in their own homes. The need for medical and nursing assessment of persons going into such care is important but as yet, no general agreement exists about who should undertake these and what should be the assessment arrangements. Warden-supervised housing units also pose difficulties. The residents of these are often very old and a high proportion are in their 80s. This produces extra strains on the warden who may have as many as a hundred old people with access to his/her services through an intercom system.

Changes in the system of benefits has allowed, over recent years, the development of increasing numbers of private rest homes and nursing homes. For those who qualify for Supplementary Benefit, the DSS will pay towards the charge of private homes. This often completely covers the amount due. Initially the registration fee for opening such an establishment was very low but is now more realistic. Supervision lies with local authorities for rest homes and district health authorities for nursing homes. Criticism has been made of the level of inspection and the standards of some of these homes. Again no assessment is made of patients entering and little is known of the subsequent movements of such patients. Certainly some move from one home to another and occasionally return to live with relatives. Medical treatment for people in private nursing homes is provided by general practitioners. Sometimes when patients move out of their home area this is difficult to obtain.

Hospital departments of geriatric medicine have also had problems and traditionally these have been of three types: maintaining adequate staffing levels of both doctors and nurses; existing in substandard accommodation; and having enough beds to meet the high demand. In many ways these have eased over the past few years. Medical staffing is easier, maybe because of the increasing number of medical graduates with an interest in geriatric medicine and more competition for posts in other specialties. The vocational training scheme for general practitioners has also helped, as a Senior House Officer post in geriatric medicine is now an encouraged option for trainees. Recruitment of nursing staff is, however, still difficult. The old workhouse type of accommodation that used to house many departments of geriatric medicine are being replaced by modern purpose-built units and these are welcome. The pressure on beds especially by long-stay patients has been eased considerably by the growth of private rest homes and nursing homes with financial help from the State, and the hospital can now discharge many patients, including those whose problems were largely associated with social-care difficulties, to these homes for continuing care. When considering old people in hospital, however, it must be remembered that only about one-third are actually in geriatric medical care and the remainder are under the care of other specialties. There is probably a need for the principles of geriatric medicine to be disseminated through the specialties if satisfactory hospital in-patient care is to be available consistently to all patients.

Finally, when considering difficulties in the provision of care it is necessary to mention co-ordination of the three major providers of this care and the need to have adequate interservice communication. The medical care of elderly people is basically the responsibility of the health services. Social services are concerned with social wellbeing. Administratively, these two partners are quite separate. The social services departments are administered by local authorities and the medical services by the Department of Health. There is a further division, however, within the medical services: hospitals and their staff are administered locally by the District Health Authority and general practitioners and their staff by autonomous Family Practitioner Committees. Despite efforts to increase co-operation by joint planning and funding, there is little to show for the effect of various reorganizations over the past decade. Co-operation on the ground between health and social workers appears to be very difficult to achieve and it is clear that social services departments have other heavy responsibilities apart from the elderly. They are burdened by financial restrictions, which result in only a very limited service being offered. Nevertheless, it is probable that the priority given to geriatric care in the community needs to be increased if proper services are to be given. There are also difficulties in providing community nursing care. These have been highlighted in the Cumberlege Report on Community Services (DHSS, 1986). The response to these difficulties will be considered later when describing nursing care. Co-operation between the service providers in the community (local authority, district health authority and Family Practitioner Committee) will eventually have to be achieved. It is possible that a single community unit providing all these services will in the end be the only way in which efficient care can be given.

As well as all these difficulties there are also changes that have been occurring in society, particularly in attitudes of families towards their elderly relatives. There is an increased expectation that high standards of professional care will be available to old people, resulting in additional pressure on community workers when these hopes and demands cannot be satisfied. Relatives and carers should, however, be supported in their search for high standards.

OVERALL AIMS OF COMMUNITY CARE FOR OLD PERSONS

Having analysed some of the difficulties that hinder the provision of a satisfactory service, the integral parts of such a service will now be described in some detail. It is, however, first necessary to define the basic aims of the care that the service should provide. The overall aim is to enable an old person to function effectively in his or her own environment. Most people want to live in their own homes so that the environment is likely to be that home. Occasionally, old people want to be in some form of sheltered care or residential home and this should be recognized.

This overall aim applies to both social and health care, and workers in both sectors should collaborate to provide the most cost-effective package of services and their resources should be carefully integrated within a geographical area so that needs are being fully met. Effective communication and co-ordination of resources is essential.

Within these overall objectives specific aims can be formulated. These are as follows:

1. To establish, when illness occurs, an accurate diagnosis on which logical treatment and an accurate prognosis can be based; this implies good day-to-day care of old people and effective management of acute diseases. Similarly, when social crises occur, effective assessment and response are needed. Often there are health and social components in an acute episode.

2. To improve, and if this is not possible, to maintain an old person's functional performance. Cure may not always be possible but an attempt should always be made to maximize effective health.

3. To enable old people to be outward-looking and to accept responsibility for caring for themselves. In this sense the provision of care itself is not the prime aim of the community worker but rather by education and encouragement to facilitate self-care amongst old persons.

4. To foster a team approach to the provision of care. This should involve both health and social workers who should form a community-care team. It is no longer acceptable that, for instance, a doctor should be involved solely in the medical aspects of old age and a social worker only in the social care. Health and social problems are inevitably interlinked and both need attention if the overall situation is to be improved. This has long been a principle of care in hospital where doctors, nurses and almoners worked in close co-operation. In the community, such co-operation is no less essential.

5. To recognize at-risk situations. Examples of these are patients living alone, the housefast, the over-75-year olds, the bereaved and those recently discharged from hospital. Special care is needed for these people.

6. To have a preventive outlook towards care. This means particularly the identification of people in need. The idea of anticipatory care has evolved in recent years. This includes primary, secondary and tertiary prevention, case finding and health promotion. There are many ways of achieving these and they will be described in Chapter 10, but the important point is the commitment to a preventive approach. This means avoiding the need for crisis intervention by forseeing how situations will evolve.

7. To provide effective continuing care for those with long-term medical problems and chronic illness. This would include maintenance therapy, surveillance and rehabilitation.

8. To provide adequate resettlement for patients who are discharged from hospital back into the community. Proper reception of patients is crucial to their continuing care.

9. To provide adequate care for dying patients, especially when they wish to die at home.

10. To establish good relationships between the community-care team for elderly patients and those providing care in hospitals or other institutions.

11. To give support and relief to informal carers who are looking after old people.

12. To provide information and education for elderly people in a neighbourhood.

13. To be prepared to be an old person's advocate in situations of difficulty.
14. To provide a responsive service both in social support and health care, with sufficient flexibility to provide, where necessary, high-intensity care as in the hospital-at-home schemes.

Some of these aims are being fulfilled very effectively. Medical care of acute illnesses and the day-to-day management of problems as they arise are probably of high standard throughout the developed world. Other aspects of care are not, however, so well performed. These include continuing care, preventive care and teamwork. These are only slowly being accepted as the norm.

RESOURCES

What resources are available in the community for the achievement of these aims? A wide range of informal and formal caring services exist.

Medical care

Medical care in the community is provided by general practitioners who may be family doctors. In the UK these are doctors who are contracted to the Family Practitioner Committee in each area. These committees are autonomous and are appointed by the DOH. They are responsible for general medical services, general dental services, pharmaceutical services and optician services. By the nature of their contract, GPs are independent and considered to be self-employed. Their income is derived from a mixture of capitation fees, basic practice allowance and item-of-service fees. The extra work involved in caring for elderly people is recognized by increased capitation fees being available for patients aged over 65, which is at one level, and, at a higher level, for patients who are over 75. This is neither an incentive to take on more nor a reward for work well done. General practitioners are also able to earn additional income from outside appointments including part-time hospital posts and other sessional activities. There is, however, very little private practice in the community.

If the proposals discussed in the White Paper *Working for Patients* go through, changes in the way general practice is organized will occur. Family Practitioner Committees will become smaller and have a more managerial role. Larger practices will have the option of budget holding status. From within this budget the doctors will be expected to provide a wide range of services for their patients. Smaller practices will have budgets managed by the District General Managers. General practitioners will, however, retain their independent contractor status. General practice has changed dramatically in the past two decades. There are now in the UK over 33 000 general practitioners and the average list of patients per doctor is in the region of 2200. The average list of patients would contain 328 (131 male and 197 female) patients aged over 65, 125 (41 male and 84 female) patients over 75 and 23 (5 male and 18 female) patients over 80. In inner-city and coastal areas these figures might be much higher and perhaps lower in suburban residential areas. Most doctors now work in groups or partnerships. Typically, each practice consists of three or four partners working together, caring for about 8000 patients. The average age of a GP is becoming lower and now only 13% are over 60 years old. The proportion of women GPs is rising and they make up about one-fifth of the total. The proportion of doctors who graduated at universities outside the UK has risen to 19% but may now be declining. There are about 1250 health centres in the UK and about 25% of doctors work from these. The remainder work from private surgery premises. The past twenty years have also seen major changes in education for general practice. Most undergraduate students now have periods of attachment to departments of general practice. Since 1982, approved training for general-practice principals has become mandatory. To achieve principal status it is necessary to complete two years in approved hospital posts and one year as a trainee in general practice. About one in every four of all practices is a training practice. Apart from the treatment and aftercare of illness, health promotion is increasingly an important part of the general practitioner's work, through maternal, child-welfare, cervical-cytology, well-woman and well-man clinics. More and more special facilities are being provided for elderly patients.

The primary-care team

Although not always functioning effectively, the basic unit for the provision of care in the community is the primary-care team. The doctor no longer works in isolation but is involved with both other health workers and social workers. There are many possible members of this team. They include the practice staff, other professionals working from health centres, social workers and a wide range of other involved people, such as dentists, pharmacists, chiropodists, therapists, the clergy, teachers, voluntary organizations, self-help groups and so on.

The way the team works
As has been described, there are many potential members of the primary-care team and also some disillusionment about how effective it has turned out to be. Ideally, the team should work together to achieve previously agreed objectives for the whole team. A football team's task is to win the game. At its simplest, primary care's perceived task is to solve problems which affect people in the community. There is of course more to it: the problems need identifying, preventing and anticipating; and some are not capable of being resolved and therefore continuing care is necessary. Despite criticism, the team actually does work well as a means of coping with problems and it does this in a particular way. There are in effect

three different primary-care teams. The first, sometimes called the *mega-team*, consists of everyone concerned in any way with caring for people in the community. This can include pharmacists, chiropodists, dieticians, speech therapists, physiotherapists, teachers, policemen, priests and many others, as well as health and social-service workers and practice staff. Within this group, however, there is an important nucleus of health and social workers who frequently are presented with problems and for this reason need to have close association with each other. These include the general practitioner, the district nurse, the midwife, the health visitor, the social worker and other key practice workers. This group is often called the *macro-team*. When faced with a problem, however, only two or three members of the macro- or mega-teams are usually involved. This is the crucial functional unit and is referred to as the *mini-team*. Thus, when an old person suffers from an ulcerated leg, the GP, the district nurse and the social worker may be the key persons involved and form the mini-team. When the situation is resolved this team disperses leaving perhaps one person behind to supervise continuing care. Often there is a key person who first recognizes the problem and brings the mini-team together. This person can be any member of the macro-team. This instigator usually takes up leadership of that particular mini-team. For instance, in the case of an old person who is blind and having problems with prescriptions, the instigator might be the pharmacist and the mini-team might consist of the pharmacist, the GP and a social worker. An old person may be found by the district nurse to have deteriorating mobility. She then needs to bring in a physiotherapist and perhaps even a social worker to form the mini-team to provide help to sort out this problem. At the level of the mini-team, the concept of teamwork is very effective and especially so with elderly people. It is, however, essential that each member of the macro-team should understand this principle and the specific and contributory roles of each member of the team. Leadership tends to fall on the instigating member and each team should understand that the leadership function is to do with the nature of the problem and not seniority or position within the overall team.

The practice staff

There are special provisions whereby a general practitioner can directly employ practice staff at the level of two per GP. Seventy per cent of their salary is reimbursed by the Family Practitioner Committee to the general practitioner. The members of the practice employed in this way include practice managers, medical secretaries, receptionists, practice nurses, nurse practitioners and sometimes data-handling secretaries and counsellors. This group forms a very important part of the primary-care team and they are very involved, often as the first contact person, with the patient. In a practice unit of 10 000 patients there would be one manager, six to seven whole-time equivalent secretaries and receptionists and up to three practice nurses, working from a treatment room. Nurse practitioners are not very common: they undertake more medical-type work and are often very involved with health promotion among elderly people.

Nursing services

Nursing services are provided within the practice by the practice nurse. He/she usually works from a treatment room and provides services that include injections, immunizations, dressings, blood sampling, check-up sessions for hypertension, diabetes, etc. They also assist the general practitioner with minor surgery, insertion of intrauterine devices and electrocardiograph recording. Many practice nurses have open access so that patients can bring problems directly to them. Elderly people often have a special place in the duties of a practice nurse; routine visiting and assessment may be undertaken.

Community-nursing services are provided by the district health authority. These services include community nurses (district nurses), community psychiatric nurses, nursing liaison teams, stoma nurses and other specialized nurses. Often district nurses are attached to practices. This means that although still employed by district health authorities, they devote their whole time to the patients of the practice or group and integrate with other members of the practice team. This has the advantages of allowing nurses to work in close co-operation with the general practitioner. There are, in England, 9000 whole-time equivalent district nurses and 6000 registered enrolled nurses assisting them. The number of nurses working in the community has increased over the last ten years and there are now about one-third more than there were in 1974. Within this expansion there has, however, been a shift in the mix of skills and grades. The number of nurses with a district-nurse qualification has decreased recently and is back to the level of ten years ago. In the same decade, the number of nursing auxiliaries has more than doubled.

The important Cumberlege Report (DHSS, 1986) highlighted some of the difficulties of nursing in the community. A series of weaknesses was found in the service provided despite improved training and better knowledge. The Report found that the needs of individual patients were not being identified systematically, nurses and general practitioners were not coordinating their activities, too much time was spent on collecting data, roles were set and traditional working methods tended to prevail, resulting in services becoming poorly co-ordinated. There was also concern about the overlap and duplication that existed between specialist nurses, health visitors, general practitioners and social-services departments. Cumberlege proposed the novel scheme of neighbourhood nursing services as a solution. This has advantages, but the proposals have been criticized because they would weaken the link between the general practitioner and the nursing services and thus would threaten the important principle of team care. It has been suggested by Williams and Wilson (1987) that GPs could form parallel community medical groups, servicing the same population unit as the community nursing group, and this would achieve a more united approach and maintain the team concept. Both these ideas would mean major change in the system of providing community care and entrenched professional attitudes may turn out to be too much of a stumbling block. However, such schemes are beginning to develop in several areas of the country and may eventually become the norm. An alternative that is also finding favour is that nurses employed in the practice should take over the role of community nurse. There is nothing to stop general practitioners from doing this and it would solve many team and administrative problems with benefit for the patients. The autonomy of the nurse would, however, need to be carefully guarded. Certainly as far as old persons are concerned, all the problems identified by Cumberlege are very pertinent: any improvement in the organization would be beneficial (DHSS, 1986). More detailed discussions of the principles of nursing in the community are given in Chapter 18.

Health-visitor services

Health visitors are also employed directly by the district health authority and many are attached to practices in the same way as district nurses. There are 9300 health visitors in England. The overall numbers increased gradually until 1984, but have started to decline since then. Health visitors have been traditionally concerned with health promotion and health education. Their work has been particularly directed towards children – especially the under-fives. With a background of training in nursing and midwifery they have been effective in promoting child health care. Health visitors have for many years also held a brief for well elderly people, but have in most cases failed to give this age group a high priority (Luker, 1987). Recent government statistics show that only 13% of patients visited by health visitors are over 65 years of age. Despite increasing recognition that the health-visitor service has not been meeting the needs of elderly people, the number of people visited has not increased since 1976. There are of course reasons for this: the age structure of the local population may influence the relative workload of health visitors and make visiting elderly persons more difficult; and specific guidelines about visiting the under-fives makes this task a priority. The personal preferences of individual health visitors may contribute to variation in visiting patterns. Health-visitor resources also vary by district. The recommendation of the DHSS of one health visitor per 3000 of the population, for those attached to general practices, is widely ignored. The growing importance of an anticipatory care programme for elderly people makes it necessary, as Luker (1987) points out, to re-think strategies for visiting elderly people. Realistic schemes for case finding and follow-up need to be introduced. Changes in role and education, together with a flexible policy towards old people, will probably be the development that most determines increased health-visitor involvement with old people in the future.

The physiotherapist/remedial gymnast

Traditionally, physiotherapists worked in hospital rehabilitation units. Now, however, the importance of rehabilitation once the patient has returned home has been understood and these services are more widely available in the community. Physiotherapists are usually employed by the district health authority but local-authority social services are also able to do this. Occasionally physiotherapists are employed directly by general practitioners. Physiotherapists' concerns are mainly with mobility. He/she must aim to prevent muscle deformity and wasting; moreover, muscle usage must be encouraged and loss of balance improved. The idea is to reduce poor co-ordination and enable the patient to walk unaided.

The occupational therapist

These therapists are also employed by district health authorities and sometimes by local-authority social-services departments. They are concerned with enabling the patient to cope with such tasks as dressing, undressing, eating, drinking, shaving, cooking, cleaning, toileting and personal care. They have suffered in the past from being thought to be merely teachers of handicrafts, which might relieve patients' boredom. They are, however, very essential to recovery in many cases. This is achieved by teaching patients finer movements and skilled activities that enable the patient to function in his/her environment after an illness. The therapy should start at the same time as physiotherapy and be a part of the overall rehabilitation strategy. Probably in the future, the role of physiotherapist and occupational therapist will merge into one.

The speech therapist

Speech therapists are concerned with communication and the problem is often a difficult one. It involves not only speech problems but reading, writing and sign language. The sense of touch is also explored. The work is closely related to that of the other therapists and is of equal importance. Unfortunately, speech therapists are in relatively short supply and the help of voluntary organizations is sometimes needed to continue the therapy on a long-term basis.

REHABILITATION

Rehabilitation of sick old people at home has been, until recently, a fairly neglected activity. Non-availability of appropriate therapists and poor co-operation between family doctors and other workers has been the main cause for ths deficiency. However, with increasing availability of therapists and a greater understanding of their value, rehabilitation has become an important part of community care. The aim is to restore the patient from a state of dependence back to independence and the ability to live a normal life. In the community there are two types of situation demanding rehabilitation. One is where the patient has been discharged from hospital and where procedures to restore function have been started but need to be continued at home. It is sometimes tragic to see the effects of the hard and dedicated work done in the hospital, which has enabled the person to return home, being rapidly reversed by failure to maintain the process when he/she is back in the community. The second situation is where the person is treated at home in the first place and where rehabilitation is needed to enable him/her once more to lead a normal life. In elderly people, this is particularly important because even minor illness can reduce the capacity for self-care and unless this is realized, full recovery may never take place.

Illnesses such as stroke may lead to major disablement and demand considerable rehabilitation, but conditions such as heart failure, pneumonia, bronchitis and urinary-tract infection, where the patient may be confined to bed even for a very short time, may also run risks of the patient developing muscular weakness, joint stiffening and general loss of mobility. It is important at the outset of an illness to get some idea of what the future holds. The consequences of an illness in terms of loss of ability to self-care must be remembered and assessment of the physical, mental, psychological and socio-environmental condition of the patient must be made with primary functional ability in mind. It is useful in this respect if the person's previous state and circumstances are known. Physical assessment involves general examination to determine functional ability and is concerned with such activities as feeding, washing and bathing. The patient's mental state also needs assessment. Intellectual impairment following stroke or concomitant senile dementia may reduce functional ability. Depression or anxiety may be present and many old people react to illness by losing self-confidence and respond with despair to the thought of losing independence. It is also important to discover changes in perception of body image as deterioration of this can affect functional performance. A careful look needs to be taken at the patient's home environment: the type of house he or she lives in may determine how he or she is to cope – will it suit the patient's new needs, if not, can it be adapted? The attitude of family and neighbours is also important.

Some relatives are unwilling to accept the burden of looking after a disabled old person and it might be that such antagonism will reduce the chance of effective rehabilitation.

These are the types of question that will need to be asked in order to plan physical rehabilitation. Factors need identifying that might interfere with this. Realism is essential when assessing the prospects of an old person, and only obtainable goals should be pursued. Many tasks are physically possible, but the patient may be unable to cope because of poor understanding, failing vision or lack of motivation. Cooking, for instance, may be dangerous. Rehabilitation services therefore must aim to achieve only what is feasible and consistent with the patient's abilities. To this end assessment should be an ongoing exercise and the team should monitor progress critically and be aware of changes in the general condition of the patient. Fluctuation of the degree of illness means that what can be done today may not be possible tomorrow.

Simple rehabilitation at home

Most rehabilitation needs to be undertaken by skilled and qualified workers. These include physiotherapists, occupational therapists and speech therapists. However, sometimes, when the services of these workers are not available or when the condition is not serious, the family alone, perhaps with the help of the community nurse, is faced with undertaking the patient's rehabilitation. The rehabilitation process should start as early in the illness as possible and will usually begin when the patient is in bed. Simple passive exercises for the affected limb should be undertaken with the aim particularly of avoiding contractures. Gentle massage will help the patient to feel more comfortable. Unaffected limbs and muscles must also be exercised to prevent disuse atrophy. Special care must be taken of the shoulder of a hemiplegic-stroke sufferer. It can very easily be deranged by relatives or other helpers when lifting the patient with either the hand in the axilla or holding the paralysed arm.

Speech therapy, where necessary, can also begin at this stage and the patient can be encouraged to articulate words. It may be possible to arrange for him/her to start reading or at least listening to the radio. As part of early occupational therapy, such things as knitting or jigsaw-puzzle solving may be introduced. As soon as is practicable, the patient should be encouraged to sit in a chair. This is feasible when he/she is able to sit without falling. Special attention should be given to the chair and it should have a seat with a surface parallel to the ground. The seat should be about 18 in (46 cm) from the floor. A firm back capable of support is necessary and it is essential for it to have arms. The chair must of course be stable. At home it is probably better that it should not have castors and trays are best avoided. The front legs should not have a connecting bar as this prevents the old person putting his/her feet back when rising. A sprung seat may help to gain the first degrees of lift in rising.

Once the patient is capable of sitting in the chair, passive movements should be continued and he/she can start to learn how to dress as an extension of the occupational therapy. Movements of the hands and fingers should be encouraged. The patient can sit on the edge of the bed or chair to move the feet up and down. The next stage is standing and this is sometimes difficult if balance is impaired. If this is so, expert physiotherapist help is usually required, but sometimes the relatives, given ample support, can teach the patient how to stand using perhaps the bed rail and then proceed to help with walking. The use of walking aids such as a Zimmer frame or tripod is often useful in helping old people to gain confidence. Gradually and with encouragement, patients should be able to achieve this mobility and at the end be able to manage for themselves the tasks of general care. Where there are more complicated problems of contractures, or movement is severely restricted, expert help should be obtained and, if necessary, admission into a hospital rehabilitation unit should be arranged.

Aids and appliances

The patient may need various aids and appliances (Mulley, 1988) to help him/her to regain independence, and if full recovery is impossible, these may become permanent features of the patient's life. Rehabilitation involves assessing which aids will be needed, and also teaching people how to use them. Aids are usually small, easily handled items and if the device is larger and non-portable, it is usually described as a piece of equipment. The word 'appliance' is used to describe an aid that is purposely made for the individual.

The idea of these aids is to enable a person to do something that would otherwise be difficult or impossible. Their function is to enable the person to overcome the effects of a disability and to become more independent. The aids themselves must be of the best design possible and they should be efficient. They should be cheap, but this does not mean shoddy or unattractive. Robust equipment is important, because anything that is likely to break will quickly lose the confidence of the user. Too many aids should be avoided as the confusion brought about by too much technology can be a danger.

The number of aids that have been devised is endless. Many are home-made and involve considerable ingenuity. Some useful aids are described under each basic care heading.

Toileting
To be able to use the toilet is important to a patient's self-respect. If the toilet is too low, this can be raised with a plastic seat. Rails can be placed

on either side to help with sitting and standing. If it is impossible for a person to use a pedestal toilet, a commode, bedpan or bottle may be necessary.

Washing
Washing the upper part of the body is usually no great problem but reaching the back and feet may be difficult and long-handled brushes and sponges can help. Getting in and out of the bath may be quite impossible, but some old people can manage with bath rails and a bath seat. Non-slip mats are essential in a bathroom. A shower is often useful.

Shaving and grooming
Shaving can be a problem for an old man and an electric razor with a long handle may help. For women, application of make-up may be helped by a long-handled lipstick holder. Similarly, combs and brushes can also be attached to long handles.

Dressing
It is obvious that disabled old persons should wear suitable clothes, avoiding buttons, preferably using zips and having everything fastening at the front. Tights and trousers for women are easier to put on, having the added advantage of extra protection and warmth and they may also hide artificial limbs or calipers. Shoes should be of the non-lace type. Various aids are also available for picking up items from the floor and also for putting on stockings.

Feeding
When feeding is a problem because of poor grip or lack of co-ordination of hand movements, cutlery with large handles may help; drinking may be facilitated through a straw or in a special cup that cannot be knocked over. Plates with stable, wide bases may make things easier and there are many devices for dealing with jugs and teapots. Non-slip table mats are also useful. Modified 'sporks' and plate rims can enable to hemiplegic to feed him/herself.

Mobility
Many aids are available to help with mobility. For support there are simple walking sticks, Zimmer frames, tripods and quadrapods. Wheelchairs are available either through the social services department or directly through a GP, using form no.AOF 5G. There are two types of wheelchair available – the transit pushchair and the self-propelled. Special designs also exist for amputees. Accessories are also available, such as cushions, base boards and harness. Occasionally, it is necessary to adapt the house by providing extra ramps and widening doors. Walking can also be assisted by shoe raises, surgical shoes and calipers with

toe-raising springs or inside irons and T-straps. Modifications for the house are sometimes possible and these can include installing support rails, levelling out steps and providing ramps, and widening doors. Hoists are also occasionally provided to help old people out of bed and into a wheelchair.

Household duties
There are many specially adapted cooking utensils. Split-level cookers are helpful, and electrical sockets should be at appropriate heights. A device may be attached to taps to make them easier to turn on. Long-handled brushes and dusters can aid cleaning as also can vacuum cleaners.

Communication
There is a range of devices to help communication. If a person is unable to speak clearly, a pencil and pad should be nearby. There are aids to help with writing, including, if appropriate, a typewriter. Reading can be helped by bookrests and books with large type. A telephone may be necessary and if this is needed to summon medical help urgently, the social services department may finance this. British Telecom can also advise on special telephones for the disabled and details can be found in the telephone directory. Alarm-call systems of various types may also be helpful. These can be two-way communication alarms, but occasionally the old person can have an alarm in the form of a wrist watch or pendant.

Hobbies
Many disabled old people like to continue with their hobbies. Help may be available from voluntary organizations. Gardening, for instance, may be possible using specially adapted tools.

Armchairs
Armchairs for old people should be suitable. Ideally they are comfortable, easy to get in and out of, safe and stable. It is easier for an old person to rise if the seat is reasonably high. Horizontal seats are uncomfortable and it is better to have a gentle backwards slope. The material should not be too hard and should not involve a fire risk. Cushions may give added comfort. Arm rests should not be too high and it is possibly better if they are filled. Legs need to have a wider base for increased stability. Avoid the so-called 'easy chair' – deep, low and acting as a foam trap.

Maintenance of rehabilitation

Having successfully rehabilitated an old person after an illness, especially if aids have been introduced to assist in this, it is absolutely essential to maintain some supervision. There is a considerable risk of deterioration if the stimulus of a professional worker is withdrawn too quickly. The work of several months can be lost in several weeks if the patient becomes apathetic. Some form of general supervision is therefore vital, so that any difficulties can be spotted early and the cause found and corrected. Aids and appliances must also be checked regularly.

OTHER PROFESSIONAL RESOURCES

The primary-care team in its widest sense also includes a number of other professions. Gerontological dentistry is becoming increasingly important as people keep their teeth into old age. Careful and appropriate use and fitting of dentures is important both for mastication and for cosmetic reasons. Many mouth and gum problems can also be helped by dentists. Examination of the mouth is an important part of screening. Pharmacists often provide the first professional contact for elderly people on health matters and are important for ensuring that they have an understanding of the medicines prescribed. These aspects are more fully discussed elsewhere in the book, but the importance of correct prescribing and dispensing for old people cannot be overstated. Another crucial aspect of old age is to maintain mobility and this involves special attention to feet. Chiropody care is therefore essential. Again screening should always involve foot examination and referral for appropriate care. The same applies to eye problems and the place of the optician in care for old people is again important. Correct glasses are invaluable. The role of teachers in the care of old people may appear to be minimal. However, it is becoming increasingly evident that old people need educational opportunities, not only with regard to health but also in leisure activities, hobbies and other interests. Professional teaching advice and encouragement will be essential if the opportunities in old age are to be maximized. Ministers of religion continue to be valued by elderly people. This is particularly true during times of illness and bereavement. They are, however, very involved in support at other times and are very helpful members of the primary-care team.

VOLUNTARY SERVICES

There is a wide range of voluntary organizations that provide help for old people. Some are concerned with the overall issues of old age and others with specific aspects of it. Of the former, Age Concern and Help the Aged are probably the best known. Their function is to campaign in the interests of old people, research into their needs and provide local and national services to help elderly people. They have also become important in raising public awareness of the problems and in furthering education and preventive activities. Other organizations concentrate on specific aspects, for instance Alzheimer's Disease Society, and The Heart, Stroke and Lung Society.

Another important group of voluntary organizations are the self-help groups. There are several hundred of these groups in the UK. Some are nationwide, others are local initiatives. Many are associated with problems experienced by elderly people. They may be disease specific, for instance Parkinson's Disease Society with 150 branches, or of a more general nature such as retirement workshops. The aim is to provide opportunities for patients and carers to meet others with similar problems and foster mutual support activities. They fulfil a valuable service and community workers should be aware of the groups in a district.

THE PRIME CARERS

The most important members of the caring team are the informal or prime carers. Usually, although not always, these carers are members of the family. Family members can include spouses, children, siblings or grandchildren. Sometimes the old person lives with relatives in a house that is not the original home. When an old person lives alone the family is occasionally some distance away and the prime carer then turns out to be a neighbour or friend. Occasionally lodgers are the only help around. The part played by the family and others in the care of old people has come to be appreciated more and more since early research by Townsend in the 1960s first demonstrated their importance (e.g. Townsend and Wedderburn, 1965). He found that all aspects of care, including nursing, housework, cooking and shopping, were undertaken by these helpers even when acute illness was not present. Quite a substantial proportion of carers also relied in times of their charge's illness on help from other relatives. Townsend found too that there were limits to family care. Thirty per cent of old people were imposing significant strains on relatives. Amongst married couples, the wife or husband provided care for the sick partner, but this also produced considerable strain on the one providing the care. There is no reason to believe that the situation is any different today and could well be worse.

The situation is often compounded by the nature of the help provided. Very often personal bodily care is required and an old person may be very modest in this respect. Some old people refuse to allow anyone else except their spouse to wash or bath them and this is especially true of men. It is thought improper for another female relative to attend to the bodily functions of an old man. Children may stop short of undertaking such tasks and this produces limitations on what can be done by the family. Old women are in a better position because it is often acceptable for a daughter to attend to her needs but sometimes this means that one member of the family is singled out for more than her fair share of the burden, because an old person will accept no-one else. This leads to an unequal distribution of responsibility for care and to breakdowns. It is often, therefore, that family help falters when attending to personal needs. This may not always be perceived because domestic tasks may continue to be undertaken very effectively.

Evidence for many of the difficulties experienced by carers has come from a study by D.A. Jones (1986), which sought to explore the network of informal and formal care available to frail elderly people, the problems of morbidity of informal carers who assist and support dependent elderly people in the community and to examine the implications of these problems on personal health and social services. The study suggests that families are caring for dependants at great cost to themselves and furthermore, that most of them are wanting to continue their caring role despite its demands. However, they need and would like more assistance from the formal community services in supporting their activities. The great majority of the carers studied were required to give personal assistance to their ageing relative and had to do this on their own. This involved assisting with personal tasks and in particular, with incontinence. Disturbed nights and dangerous behaviour, particularly falling, were aspects of caring that caused most distress to carers. The study suggested that those caring for an elderly person cannot draw upon a large network of informal or formal carers that had previously been thought to be the case. This was particularly so if the carer was living with the elderly person. In that case they had largely to bear the burden of care on their own with little support from services or other relatives. A quarter of the sample of carers perceived their health as being affected by their caring role. A quarter reported that their social life had been impaired as a result of acting as a carer. The lack of privacy and personal freedom affected their family life. A quarter of the carers had not had a holiday for five years and one-tenth of the sample reported that they had ceased employment in order to care for their dependent elderly relative. An unbearable amount of stress as a consequence of caring was reported by almost one-fifth of the sample. In general, daughters seemed to suffer more hardship than other carers. This is probably because caring for dependent parents is only one of the many responsibilities facing mature women. Children and husbands also make demands on their time and emotions and this causes problems of priorities. Only a minority of the carers in the study were receiving the support of personal health and social services. For those that were, community nurses and home helps were the services most commonly visiting. Home helps and meals on wheels were much less likely to be available where a carer was living with the elderly dependent. It was thought that carers needed training in various aspects of caring and that health visitors may be the most suitable people to undertake this task. Many carers felt they needed advice on, for instance, how to cope with incontinence, how to care for dependants after a stroke and how to lift their dependants without risking their own health. Health visitors could also provide advice on benefits and attendance allowance. There was found to be an overwhelming need of respite or relief care for carers. The difficulty most often mentioned by carers was the time and the unremitting nature of caring. Regular planned predictable breaks were what they reported needing most. Night disturbance caused a great deal of distress to carers and there was an obvious need for night sitters to provide a break for those carers to enable them at least to have some unbroken nights' sleep. The belief that voluntary agencies could provide the major source of support to carers and their dependants could not be substantiated by the study. The services they provided were very much valued and appreciated, but it was felt that they could in no way be seen as the focal point for future community care. Only a minority of carers estimated to be eligible for an attendance allowance had applied for it. Many carers did not know of its existence, or if they did, did not know of the appeals system.

It seems therefore that the idea of 'community care' has only a limited application and in the majority of situations the burden of care in this particular study fell heavily on one individual with very little support from other family members or community services. It is clear therefore that if families are going to continue to provide substantial support for the elderly population to enable them to live in the community rather than in institutions they will need to be supported by community services in order to maintain a reasonable quality of life. Future policies concerning the care of elderly people need to be family orientated, not individual orientated; innovations are required to support the family as a whole.

The Association of Carers

The Association of Carers is a national body that concerns itself with the needs of carers. It encourages the formation of local groups where carers with mutual problems can provide each other with help and support. An advice service is available and information can be obtained very easily. As a national organization it hopes to improve awareness of the carer's contribution and if necessary, to change the system. Full details can be obtained from The Association of Carers, 58 New Road, Chatham, Kent, ME4 4QR.

SECONDARY CARE

Secondary care is provided by the District Health Authorities through their hospital and consultant services. These services reach out into the community in a number of different ways.

Out-patient departments

These are important links between primary and secondary care and do not involve a patient being admitted to hospital. A patient's attendance at an out-patient department depends on the GP referring the patient to a consultant. The consultant may return the patient to GP care or continue to review the situation at the out-patient clinic. Often shared care is arranged between the two doctors. It is possible for the patient to receive other services within the hospital, for instance physiotherapy, speech therapy and certain special investigations that might be necessary. Rehabilitation after hospital in-patient treatment is often arranged in this way.

Domiciliary visit

A consultant may undertake a visit to the patient's home for assessment and opinion. This is initiated by the GP, who ideally will also be present at the interview. It is used when a patient is not well enough to travel and also allows the consultant to see the patient at home and assess how he/she is coping at home. In these circumstances the consultant becomes a member of the primary-care team. Often hospital admission is avoided in these circumstances, both the family and the GP being reassured.

Geriatric community-liaison team

A team of nurses based in the hospital is available in some areas to visit patients in their own homes after discharge from hospital. They offer support and advice, particularly to relatives. The function is very much one of liaison between the hospital and carers in the community. Supervision of the rehabilitation and continuing care of patients is very much part of this work. They can also involve special visits for those on a waiting list for admission to hospital.

Day hospital

Most geriatric services now provide day-hospital facilities. The main purpose of this is to continue rehabilitation and maintain progress previously made in the hospital. The day hospital also provides services for patients who have not been in hospital. The patients spend most of the day there and usually transport is arranged both there and back by ambulance. Relief is provided for the relatives in this way. Medical and nursing services are available on the spot and if necessary, admission or re-admission can be arranged. Early discharge from hospital is often facilitated. It is vital that the GP be fully informed as to treatment and especially the drugs that are being prescribed because it is the GP who is responsible for the patient when he or she is at home. There is a risk of mistakes being made when two doctors are responsible for the same patient. Treatment cards kept with the patient are important in these circumstances.

NEW PROPOSALS

The White Paper *Working for Patients* outlines plans for hospitals to opt for self-governing status. The impact of these proposals in the care of the elderly remains to be seen. Economic pressures may mean that old people are not given high priority with a resultant reduction in geriatric services. This may mean more travelling for elderly patients.

REFERENCES

DHSS (1986) Cumberlege Report, Department of Health and Social Security. *Neighbourhood Nursing – focus for care. Report of the Community Nursing Review*, HMSO, London.

Jones, D.A. (1986) *A Survey of Carers of Elderly Dependants Living in the Community. Final Report.* Research Team for the Care of the Elderly, University College of Wales College of Medicine, Cardiff.

Luker, K.A. (1987) Health visitor involvement with the elderly, in *Preventive Care of the Elderly: a review of current developments* (Eds R.C. Taylor and E.G. Buckley), Royal College of General Practitioners, London, Occasional Paper 35, pp. 42–4.

Mulley, G. (Ed.) (1988) Everyday aids and appliances. Series in *Br. Med. J.*, **296**, 2 January–7 May.

Opit, L.J. (1977) Domiciliary care for the elderly sick. Economical neglect? *Br. Med. J.*, **1**, 30–3.

Townsend, P. and Wedderburn, D. (1965) *The Aged in the Welfare State*, Bell, London.

Williams, E.I. and Wilson, A.D. (1987) Health care units: an extended alternative to the Cumberlege proposals. *J. R. Coll. Gen. Pract.*, **37**, 507–9.

9 Social-care resources

Most advanced countries have community-welfare services, but they sometimes differ in form and emphasis. Many European countries, such as Denmark and Sweden, have a long history of social care for people, and a wide variety of services is usually available. In the USA such care was started much later and was mainly centred on institutions. Self-help has always been a strong life philosophy in the USA, but recently community-based services have been developed to help the aged. In the Soviet Union a full range of services is provided, with particular emphasis on prevention of problems and rehabilitation of old people back into the community. In the UK a comprehensive service is provided for old persons. Help is available from local authorities through their social-services departments. Financial help is available from Central Government through the DSS. In addition to this a considerable amount of help is also given by voluntary and religious organizations. Although the private sector is mainly involved in residential care, it is likely to contribute more in the future to general social-care resources.

The recently published (1988) Griffiths Report, *Community Care: Agenda for Action*, is an important document that contains wide-ranging proposals for community care in the UK that could change provisions quite dramatically. How far these proposals will be implemented remains to be seen. The Report calls upon the Government to make a clear statement of its community-care objectives and priorities. Local social-service authorities are charged with assessing the care needs of the community and individuals. When organizing delivery of packages of care, they should make maximum use of the voluntary and private sectors to widen consumer choice. The effect of this will be to enlarge considerably the local authorities' responsibilities in this area. The Report further makes important points about health matters. It recommends that health authorities should continue to be responsible for medically required community-health services, including making any necessary input into assessing needs. It also recommends that general medical practitioners should be responsible for ensuring the local social service authorities are aware of their patients' needs for non-health care. Although doctors already undertake this task, it marks a change in policy by giving them specific responsiblities.

SOCIAL SERVICES

The provision of social services for needy old people has been established in the UK for a considerable time as part of the package available under the old Poor Law provisions. Since World War II it has been consistent government policy to enable old people, if they wished, to continue living at home for as long as possible. To this end legislation has been enacted to allow local authorities to provide supporting services. The *National Assistance Act* of 1948 required local authorities to provide residential accommodation for persons who, by reasons of age, infirmity or any other circumstance, are in need of care and attention, which is not otherwise available to them. The *Chronic Sick and Disabled Persons Act* of 1970 and Section 45 of the *Public Health Act* in 1968 gave local authorities power to act to help old people in the community. The *Local Authority Social Services Act* in 1970 formalized many of the services being provided and brought into being the unified local-authority social services departments.

Social services departments have now been in existence for nearly twenty years and their record in promoting the welfare of the people has been variable. Intentions have always been good, but many difficulties have been encountered. The further reorganization of local government, which brought new authorities into being on 1 April 1974, delayed development of some initiatives because of resultant management changes and redistribution of boundaries. It was hoped that having the same boundaries with health authorities would make communication between health and social workers easier. Unfortunately, this has not been helped by more recent organization, which has sacrificed co-terminosity. Problems of finance and manpower were additional reasons for failure to achieve objectives and these matters have not yet been resolved.

Certain aims and philosophies have, however, been developed. It has emerged that the primary concern of social workers is not so much the provision of services, but more the recognition of social problems. By doing this it is hoped that professional intervention will enable the problem, once recognized, to be resolved, and hence allow the family to remain independent in the community and function without support. If this fails, ongoing support services would be necessary to enable the person to continue to lead as full and satisfying a life as possible. A further concern is to prevent social distress by early prevention, and to use skilful preventive measures in the community. It is, however, important to remember that most direct work with elderly people and their families in the community is carried out not by social workers who are increasingly wholly engaged in child-care work, but by domiciliary services/home-help organizers and social-work assistants. It is helpful that the value system of these personnel is more geared to practical support and taken overall, resources for elderly people in the community from social service departments are primarily practical, for instance home help, aids and adaptions, meals on wheels and day care.

Although there are national guidelines for levels of staff employed by local-authority social services departments, there is great variation in the extent to which they meet these guidelines. Some authorities exceed the norm but others fall far short. In the case of home helps, for instance, the average level is little over half the recommended figure, although this has improved marginally over the years.

The General Household Survey (OPCS, 1986) details the use of personal and social services by sex and age (see Table 9.1). It will be seen that overall the level of these services is not high. Home-help usage increases with age but it is surprising that in the 85-plus age group the uptake of meals on wheels, lunch clubs and day-centre places decreases. This is probably because this age group has this need met either in residential homes or by active primary carers. There is evidence that the level of support services is influenced by mental health of elderly persons, and this is especially so for chiropody, community nursing, home help and meals on wheels. Mentally affected patients use these services significantly more.

The range of possible services will now be described. Information about what there is locally can be obtained centrally in England and Wales from the DSS or in Scotland from the Social Work Department of the Scottish Office.

Home help

In 1984, home-help services were used by 10% of all over-65-year-old elderly in Great Britain (OPCS ,1986). The service entitles an old person to receive help in the house of domestic nature, usually for two to three hours per day for any number of days of the week. The service has evolved over the past few years and a very flexible approach is now usually available. In some authorities, home helps are now termed 'community care assistants' in line with new national agreements on conditions of service and a new job description, which includes personal care to clients. Very careful assessment is made of a patient's need and note is made of the critical points of the day and night when help is required, and also what type of help it should be. However, within this flexibility it is the intention that the work undertaken is that which is beyond the capability of the old person. General cleaning, tidying, shopping and cooking are included. The visit also provides interesting company for the old person, which relieves loneliness and acts as a contact with the outside world and particularly the social services department itself. The availability of home-help services is limited and is probably not enough to

Table 9.1 Use of some personal social services by elderly people in the month before interview, by sex and age, persons aged 65 and over, Great Britain, 1984

Personal social services	Age					
	65–69	70–74	75–79	80–84	85 and over	All 65 and over
			Percentage who used service			
Home help						
Men	2	4	9	14	25	6
Women	4	6	14	29	33	12
All elderly	3	5	12	24	31	10
Meals on wheels						
Men	1	1	4	10	6	3
Women	1	1	3	10	5	3
All elderly	1	1	4	10	5	3
Lunch out*						
Men	2	2	4	2	4	3
Women	8	2	4	11	7	4
All elderly	2	2	4	8	6	4
Lunch provided[†]						
Men	2	3	8	12	8	5
Women	3	3	7	17	12	7
All elderly	3	3	7	15	11	6
Day centre						
Men	2	2	5	4	3	3
Women	4	5	7	10	9	6
All elderly	3	4	6	8	7	5
Bases = 100%						
Men	492	480	315	163	71	1521
Women	597	667	502	287	186	2239
All elderly	1089	1147	817	450	257	3760

* At lunch club or day centre.
[†] Includes meals on wheels and lunch out.

Source: OPCS (1986)

satisfy the needs of the population (Norman, 1982). Actual allocations to individuals are relatively low, rarely more than four hours per week, and do not appear to increase very significantly with greater dependence. The financial arrangements are flexible and vary from place to place. Some authorities provide a free service, on the grounds that the deserving will not then be afraid to ask. Other authorities make a charge based on a means test. The person's resources are assessed by the local home-help organizer at the same time as the need for assistance.

Meals on wheels

About 3% of elderly people over 65 receive meals on wheels (OPCS, 1986). Over 26 million meals are delivered annually in England to elderly people in their own homes. Half of these are delivered by voluntary organizations; this accounts for more than two-thirds of all meals served. The highest proportion of these meals is served to people of 80 years and over. The old person is usually provided with a hot meal on two or three days a week. This is usually not quite enough to meet their requirements. The nutritional value of this meal is good and although the old person has to pay, the service is subsidized, usually by the local authority. In some areas the extent of the service is widened to provide meals at other times of the day and at weekends. An emergency meals-on-wheels service is also sometimes available.

Luncheon clubs

The number of meals served in luncheon clubs has gone down between 1976 and 1986 from 16 million to 13 million per year (DHSS, 1987). In contrast, the number of meals on wheels served has increased. Luncheons are provided at centres often located in community homes or church halls. The service is primarily used by old people sufficiently mobile to get out of the house and who can become involved in a little social activity. It has the advantage of efficiency so that more old people can be catered for. The meal is supervised by a responsible person who, as a secondary objective, can keep an eye on the group and detect any signs of deterioration.

Day centres and day care

These are of two types. A day centre may be a meeting place where old people can attend to see friends and engage in social activities. Hobbies can be catered for and there may be the opportunity for games and craft work. Sometimes the centre is in the form of a workshop where old people can come for certain hours during the day and earn money. A different type of centre is where day care is provided. Here, full residential care is available for the day time and the centre is often associated with a residential home. Full supervision is present and meals are given. The type of person attending is usually dependent on some form of care, particularly if he or she lives alone or the family are unable to provide care throughout the day. Transport is often provided for old people to get to and from these centres. This type of care is also useful in providing an intermediate stage between residential accommodation and the patient's own home. It allows flexibility to be achieved between levels of care.

RESIDENTIAL CARE

Part III of the *National Assistance Act* of 1948 required local authorities to provide residential care for elderly persons, hence the term 'Part III accommodation'. Homes can be run either by the local authority itself or by sponsorship in voluntary or privately owned homes. Initially the homes were seen to be hotel-type lodgings for fit old people, but it is now regarded as preferable to keep this type of person in their own home for as long as possible. Residential care on a permanent basis is now provided only where a person cannot manage at home or in the community even with domiciliary support, provided that hospital care is not needed. As has been described earlier, there has been a major change in the provision of residential accommodation for old people during the past decade. The dramatic increase in the numbers of private rest homes and nursing homes has meant the number of places available in local authorities has slightly decreased. The overall effect is that a greater proportion of elderly people than ever is accommodated in residential care or nursing home. This is in effect an important policy decision taken by default and without public debate.

In general, the person admitted to Part III homes should be one who is reasonably well and mobile, as the homes are not intended to provide nursing care. The patient should be able to use a toilet, attend for meals, dress and have enough mobility to walk to the bedroom, albeit aided by a Zimmer frame. These days it is usually the more frail who are admitted to residential accommodation. Some degree of disability is usually present and minor nursing attention may be needed. There have always been people with mild degrees of mental impairment in residential homes, but care must be taken not to include too many of these as an unfavourable environment may be created for the more lucid residents. Some areas have homes which cater only for elderly mentally infirm patients. Assessment of a person for admission to a residential home is therefore important and a discussion of assessment is included in Chapter 14. People are often admitted to welfare homes from their own home in the community, but a sizeable proportion, probably about half, are admitted direct from hospital. Ideally, an assessment should take place before admission, but sometimes because of an emergency situation this is not possible. It should, nevertheless, take place as soon as convenient thereafter. The decision to admit an old person to a home is taken by the local authority social workers, often on no grounds other than social incompetence without medical assessment, the ultimate responsibility being with the director of the department of social services. The decision is not always easy, and balancing the degree of care needed with what can be provided at home, and the best interests of the old person is sometimes a fine one. It often means balancing gains and losses which the individual concerned should consider very carefully.

The health of the old person is often a crucial factor when admission to a residential home is considered and, as has been mentioned, this is where assessment is helpful. It should be multidisciplinary and include a health assessment by a doctor with experience of working with old people. It is very disappointing that agreement has not been reached by the British Geriatric Society, the Royal College of General Practitioners and the Royal College of Psychiatrists for a joint initiative in agreeing guidelines. Separate statements giving advice have, however, been issued by all three of these bodies. These are essentially the same except when it comes to what type of doctor (e.g. consultant geriatrician, consultant psychiatrist and GP) should undertake the assessment. Clearly each group has a vested interest. It is probable that such an assessment could be undertaken by a doctor who is experienced in caring for elderly patients and this could include all these types of doctor. As Brocklehurst *et al.* (1978) have shown, there is real concern that old people are sometimes inappropriately admitted to welfare homes. General guidelines on assessment are given in Chapter 14, but it is important when admission to homes is considered that the following should be observed:

1. that appropriate and ongoing medical care is fully available to patients in the home;
2. that medical advice is available to social services departments at the point of admission so that assessment of need is genuinely multidisciplinary;
3. that full consideration is given during assessment to the possibility of alternative means of care – in hospital, sheltered housing or very sheltered housing and to consider what support services would be required if the client were to remain in his/her own home;
4. that general advice is available to the staff of a home about the nature and level of medical-care provisions;
5. that arrangements are made for occasional reassessments of the residents' needs and placement.

These guidelines apply equally well to private rest homes and nursing homes, which are described in the next section.

Once an old person enters a local authority home on a permanent basis this then becomes his or her residence with built–in security of tenure. The old person can stay there until he/she dies or is admitted to hospital. Financial arrangements will vary and depend upon an old person's resources and income. This also needs careful discussion before final arrangements are made with both the prospective resident and the family as often it involves selling the old person's home. Sometimes a trial period is helpful before permanent decisions are taken.

Sometimes, but not often, an old person who has been in residential accommodation achieves a substantial recovery and can once again sustain an independent life in the community. When this happens, because that person is occupying a residential place that is in heavy demand, the local authority departments of social services and housing will sometimes co-operate to find a fresh home for the person concerned, probably in a sheltered housing unit. However, in reality, if a person has given up their home in the community it is difficult to persuade housing authorities to rehouse them from residential care, partly because of the increased pressures on wardens in sheltered housing.

There is a wide variety of buildings used as old people's homes. Some are modern and purpose-built, but others are converted old houses of various sizes and can even date back to the old Poor Law days. It is important that they are attractive and that the old person can identify it as home. Some authorities allow an old person to bring articles of furniture or at least sentimental pieces to decorate his/her room. The management should provide an environment in this way that enables an old person to lead as normal a life as possible. Independence with dignity is vitally necessary for the wellbeing of an old person and particularly so in an institution. Units where patients undertake their own cooking and laundry have been introduced successfully in many residential homes and this adds to the feeling that an old person can at least do something for him/herself. All residents should be encouraged to join in social activities outside as well as inside and take part in the running of the home. Such things as looking after their own rooms and helping in the garden might well be encouraged. How effective this is depends upon the head of the home and the staff. They are expected to provide care that is appropriate to a residential setting and equivalent to that provided by a caring relative. This may well include help with washing, bathing, toileting and care during illness, but would not involve long-term nursing care, and for this reason it is perhaps better that the head of the department should not be called matron. Nursing and medical care should be provided by the primary health-care team. Some doctors continue to look after their patients in welfare homes, but increasingly one doctor is prepared to take on the care of all residents. Privacy and confidentiality should be maintained on medical matters within the home. Other services such as those provided by the chiropodist, the optician and the dentist should be made available in the usual way. Many heads of homes are qualified nurses, but this is not necessary. The real expertise of the staff lies in the field of inter-personal relationships. A social-work qualification is valuable.

Apart from permanent residence, short-stay accommodation is often available for old people who might have some temporary domestic difficulty. Holiday relief for relatives often falls into this category. Sometimes, too, an old person benefits from a short trial stay at the home. This enables him/her to test out the idea of permanent residence and make the sometimes traumatic transition from home to welfare institution easier. Similarly, patients transferred from hospital to a welfare home will need special care and understanding in the first few weeks of adjustment.

PRIVATE NURSING HOMES AND REST HOMES

In the care of elderly people there has in recent years been an expansion of non-statutory residential establishments. The balance has changed so that the private sector is rapidly overtaking the local authorities as the main suppliers of residential care. The underlying reason for this change has been demographic changes that have resulted in a population of elderly people that is larger than ever before. It was known that this would happen but there was little preparation. Local authorities have been unable to cope with the demands and the private sector has eagerly entered the field to cater for a growing market. The government has helped, possibly unintentionally, by providing Social Security funds to support residence in private homes. There are two types of these homes: private nursing homes and rest homes. The former cater for a wide variety of patients including the post-operative convalescent, the chronic sick and the terminally ill, but are nevertheless largely devoted to elderly people. Nursing facilities are available in these homes and staff include fully trained nurses. This type of home must be registered with the District Health Authority. Rest homes, on the other hand, provide residential care for old people but do not provide any nursing facilities. Rest homes have to be registered with local authorities. There is some blurring in the precise differences between nursing homes and rest homes and some have dual registration.

Between 1980 and 1984 nearly 6000 additional nursing-home places were added, and 300 new private nursing homes and hospitals were opened, with an increase in bed capacity of 17%. In 1985 there were over 33 000 beds for elderly people. The persons in these nursing homes are usually more dependent than people living in residential homes, but there is some overlap. Rest homes for elderly people provided by the private sector have increased at a very rapid rate. In England there were about 32 000 private places in 1979, but by December 1984 there were an estimated 77 000 places. This represents an increase of about 140% in just under five years. It is possible that the rate of growth has decreased and perhaps the market is now being satisfied. High property values, particularly in the south of England, have probably contributed to this slow down. There is also uncertainty as to the continued level of DSS benefit support. It is possible that if this is reduced or abolished, there will be a major emergency in the supply of residential care for old people.

Much of the increase in the first years of both nursing homes and rest homes took place in an atmosphere of legal confusion. The 1984 *Residential Homes Act*, however, consolidated and extended the existing law. More elaborate registration and inspection regulations were introduced and the registration fee was increased substantially. Guidelines were introduced as to the type of provision that should be provided. For instance, in rest homes there is an emphasis on single rooms, private space, personal dignity and control by the patients of their own money and drugs. In nursing homes the guidelines dealt with the provision of trained staff and procedures for the control of medication. Little was said, however, about the provision of personal space. A major problem has occurred because of the possibility of dual registration. It has meant that there has been difficulty, because of the different guidelines for each type of establishment, in providing effective facilities for both types of patient, that is, those who need nursing and those who need a degree of autonomy and space. This has meant some concern about the quality of care in dually registered establishments. Enlightened experiments are, however, taking place and it may be possible to resolve some of these issues.

Another problem has been the provision of medical cover to these establishments. Normally this is provided by a general practitioner. Sometimes patients come from a distance to take up residence in a home and have no local GP. In these circumstances, it is possibly better that one GP looks after all patients in a particular establishment. Sometimes special arrangements have to be made for this by the home, a local practice and the FPC. The question arises as a whether a general practitioner should receive a retainer for duties carried out within a private nursing home. The General Medical Services Committee of the BMA has given guidelines on duties for which such reimbursement can be accepted. They include advice on general management involving such things as arrangements for storing drugs, disposal of clinical waste, patient record systems, confidentiality and medico-legal matters. Also included is advice regarding staff appointments and training, and the provision of an occupational health service. Patients who do not wish to receive NHS provision can be treated on a private basis.

Clearly, there are problems yet to be solved in the private sector. Assessment of residents at admission needs to be undertaken and professional support and advice needs to be available to both types of home from local authorities and health authorities. An efficient inspection procedure is important. Provision also needs to be made for training of staff and this should be taken into account by the registering authorities. Finally, the establishment of national guidelines for standards of care would help because of the differing expectations that exist between local authorities and health authorities both locally and nationally. Local flexibility is, however, important and homes should be sensitive to neighbourhood needs.

SHELTERED ACCOMMODATION

The provision of sheltered accommodation for old people has also been a development of recent years. Accommodation is usually provided by local-authority housing departments, but sometimes by housing associations. The units can be of a bungalow type, but also may be two- or three-storey blocks of flats. An average of about 36 dwellings would constitute a unit together with a warden to supervise. Sometimes there are communal-eating and meeting facilities and laundering. Living in these sheltered units can provide certain advantages such as cheap TV licence rates. Many have intercom and alarm-bell systems. Units with these latter facilities are best used to meet the needs of less-active elderly people. The warden's job is basically that of a good neighbour who will summon the assistance of other services and relatives if necessary. He/she is not expected to do any nursing or give domestic help, but more to check that individuals are coping and not developing illnesses or being neglected.

On occasions, sheltered-housing units have been built near a Part III residential home, thus enabling the tenants to receive the benefit of support and attention from the highly qualified staff of the residential home, and yet maintain a more satisfying state of independence. If increasing age brings about a general deterioration, then the move into the residential home can be far less traumatic than is often the case.

HOUSING ASSOCIATIONS

Housing associations or trusts were first established in the early part of this century as charitable bodies, to cater for those with special housing needs, including elderly people. Larger national associations such as the Anchor Housing Association and the Hanover Housing Association cater specially for the housing needs of old people. There are variations in the type of accommodation provided, some schemes involving groups of flats, or, as in the case of the Anchor Association, the objective being to provide warden-supported sheltered housing. There is a growth of sheltered housing with extra care run by housing associations. These are built to special standards with extra care staff on the premises in addition to a warden. Some societies, such as Abbeyfield, aim to provide elderly people with their own rooms within the security and companionship of small households. All are registered charities and non-profit-making bodies. Legislation exists to promote and regulate the housing-association movement.

ADDITIONAL SERVICES

Laundry services

Most local authorities provide a laundry service to assist those caring for old people, particularly if incontinence is a problem. This is usually free. Special incontinence pads and equipment are also available through the community nursing services.

Extra heating, extra diet, help with transport fares

Local authorities through their social services departments may provide additional heating for an old person's house if this is considered necessary. Also, in some parts of the country help is available for extra dietary needs and in some cases, concessionary bus fares are available for old people. Finance is usually arranged through the local authority. Sometimes help is available with telephones where this is necessary. Holidays, too, are occasionally arranged.

Adaptations of houses

These can be arranged by the social services department if they are considered necessary to help the old person; for example, help may be obtained in installing lifts or shower units, and in the widening of doorways to take a wheelchair.

Aids and appliances

These are provided by the social services department and are specially helpful where rehabilitation is necessary (see Chapter 8).

Blind register

Social services departments are particularly interested in blind people. They keep a blind register and offer special services for elderly blind people.

SOCIAL CASEWORK

The nature and extent of social casework that may be undertaken among elderly people can only briefly be touched upon here. It has been said that the social problems experienced by old people are practical rather than emotional, at least on the surface, and it is physical help that is needed rather than supportive casework. However, this is debatable and it is likely that old people experience the full range of emotional problems and help may be needed by them or their families to manage these difficulties. Sometimes specific groups in a community, for instance old people living in sheltered housing, may need social support to smooth out the interpersonal differences that may occur. An obvious example when people live in a close community is rivalry for friendship or subgroup formation. Sometimes an old person may be excluded from social intercourse for reasons that are at first not clear. These types of problem involve deep analysis and attempts to restore social balance are often very time-consuming. Long-term support may be necessary and this can some-times be achieved by using group activity, especially at day centres. Rehabilitation of patients discharged from hospital or welfare homes can also be helped by these means.

Social workers can also help to develop the community's awareness of the problems of old people. They can create 'good neighbour' schemes and identify trouble spots where perhaps an area consisting of a high proportion of elderly residents is being persistently vandalized. The aim in these circumstances is to make the community socially self-supporting. The work involves some subtlety and it is important to avoid segregating elderly people from the rest of the community. Integration is the principal objective.

REFERENCES

Brocklehurst, J.C., Carty, M.H., Leeming, J.T. and Robinson, J.A.M. (1978) Medical screening of old people accepted for residential care. *Lancet*, **ii**, 141–2.

DHSS (1987) *Health and Personal Social Services Statistics for England*, HMSO, London.

Griffiths Report (1988) *Community Care: Agenda for Action. A report to the Secretary of State for Social Services by Sir Roy Griffiths*, HMSO, London.

Norman, A. (1982) *Home Help: Key Issues in Service Provision*, Centre for Policy in Ageing, London.

OPCS (1986) *General Household Survey, 1984*, HMSO, London.

10 *Preventive and anticipatory care*

Medical care in the community has, over a long period, been provided by family doctors. In the past this care was usually initiated by a patient's request for help, either by way of a consultation, or a request for a home visit. This is the so called 'reactive' form of response. The aim of the doctor was to respond promptly and relieve the acute situation, the emphasis being on cure. Thus, most general-practitioner care was episodic, but because of the doctor's ready availability it was generally successful in dealing with immediate problems.

This reactive response was also the norm when providing for care for old people. It was, however, appreciated that there were limitations in concentrating on cure alone when dealing with elderly people and it was necessary to have an eye on long-term problems. There developed, therefore, the custom of regular visiting that was an acknowledgement of both this and the fact that old people needed surveillance if therapy was to be effectively monitored, deterioration detected early and new problems identified. Unfortunately the decision as to which particular patients were to receive these visits, especially in pre-National Health Service days was made in rather an arbitrary fashion, often depending on the patient's ability to pay. Such visits ran the risk of becoming merely social encounters with little medical content. Even so, these were doctor-initiated actions in the so-called 'pro-active' mode and were valuable in that interest was shown and contact made.

Regular visiting has been maintained as part of modern general practice: indeed over half doctor–patient contacts in the over-85 age group take place in the patient's home. There has, however, developed an increasing realization that it is often the wrong patients who are being visited. Those in real need are often not accurately identified and with the increased numbers of old people, the policy of visiting all old patients has become impractical. The average number of people over 75 years old on an average GP's list is over 125. A GP would need to undertake at least 30 visits per week to achieve a monthly visit for each patient. Furthermore, such visits in most cases would be unnecessary because most of this age group would be well and many could attend the surgery. Nevertheless, the concept of keeping an eye on elderly patients was good and is still applicable. There has therefore developed over the past two decades a range of alternatives to the practice of regular visiting.

DEFINITIONS

Before going on to describe the various methods that have been evolved, it is necessary to make some definitions. In some senses the whole area has become confused by terminology. There is an overlap in meaning between some of the terms used.

Prevention.   This means what it says: to keep off harmful effects, which in the case of elderly people means avoiding disease if possible and if not, at least treating it early so that it can be contained. The prime aim is to prevent loss of function.
Primary prevention.   This means stopping the disease before it has had a chance to arise: an example would be immunization against influenza.
Secondary prevention.   This means detection of disease at an early or pre-cursor state when it is actually curable and often asymptomatic. Examples would include cervical cytology and routine breast screening.
Tertiary prevention.   This means the early recognition of established disease so that treatment can be initiated at such a stage that alleviation of suffering and preservation of function may be achieved, although cure may not be possible. Most of the formal screening processes involving old patients are of this tertiary type.
Case finding.   This is where some of the confusion has occurred. Case finding is essentially the same as tertiary prevention – early recognition of existing disease or loss of function. Williamson (1987) stresses that screening for loss of function is an integral part of case finding and teaches that the search for it should occur in four equally important areas:

1. loss of physical function
2. loss of mental function
3. loss of social function
4. loss of family function.

This widening of the idea to include, for instance, carer problems is very significant. Tertiary screening of course implies formal screening of an entire population, for instance the over-75-year olds in a practice at the initiation of the *doctor*. Case finding, on the other hand, refers to detection of problems opportunistically during contacts initiated by *patients* as well as during more formal routine surveillance. The difference between the two terms therefore lies in how the preventive care is organized. Case finding is essentially a two stage exercise. The first stage identifies patients with problems and can be undertaken in several different ways. This is then followed by the second stage which is the referral onwards of patients found to have problems for further assessment.

Disease prevention.   This term is a widely embracing one often used in America. It encompasses primary, secondary and tertiary prevention as outlined previously.

Health promotion.   This term again has a wide meaning. It embraces all forms of health education, sensible living, exercise, diet, avoidance of smoking, alcohol temperance and so on. It is also concerned with the important aspect of self-help, especially in the case of elderly people.

Anticipatory care.   This term is used to describe the process of opportunistic case finding where there is some positive health promotion at the same time. It is therefore a composite term to describe health promotion and disease prevention at normal doctor – patient contact. The process can also be undertaken by other health workers, for instance district nurses, health visitors and practice nurses, and, in a social sense, by social workers.

Assessment.   Again there is some overlap because assessment is sometimes used as synonomous with screening. However, assessment is really a wide term that describes what happens at various times and in various situations when an old person has health and social status examined. There are many different reasons for doing full assessment and these are described in Chapter 14.

DEVELOPMENT OF PREVENTIVE AND ANTICIPATORY CARE

The idea of a preventive approach to problems of old age goes back nearly forty years. The beginning was dominated by geriatric-consultant screening clinics, the most famous being at Rutherglen in Scotland where Cowan and Anderson (1952) assessed patients referred by general practitioners in an attempt to identify illness at an early age. This was tertiary prevention aimed to effect a cure if possible, but otherwise alleviation of the problem. However, it was James Williamson *et al.* (1964) who gave real impetus to the idea of this type of prevention by describing the phenomenon of 'unreported need'. This stimulated the interest of general practitioners and some responded by introducing comprehensive screening of elderly people into their practices. During this period, mainly in the early 1970s, Williams *et al.* (1972) introduced the concept of 'effective health' with an emphasis on functional ability. His early studies concentrating on the over-75-year-old age group gave the first clue that problems associated with ageing may not start until well beyond the normal retiring age. Much of this early screening work was important for gaining an understanding of the natural history of old age in the community. The significance of unreported need was developed and a process described that could be set down as a *dynamic equation*: multiple pathology together with failure to report symptoms results in loss of function. This can be described as "the Law of Diminishing Function". Fortunately the equation is reversible. Ageing was set into a highly variable longitudinal perspective and this underlined the value of primary-care research.

By about 1974, however, it became clear that full comprehensive screening was impractical and doubt was also cast on its value. Follow-up studies in general practice showed that enormous effort was being expended by the doctor without convincing evidence of the benefits to health. A study that examined the value of such screening in middle age was published in 1977 and because of its negative findings had an important effect on attitudes towards screening in general (The South-East London Screening Study Group, 1977). The conclusions of this study were often extended, probably wrongly, to older age groups. The result was that comprehensive screening went out of favour.

This led to a more selective approach, the assumption being that some of the elderly needed such care more than others. Taylor, Ford and Barber (1983) examined patients from previously identified at-risk groups with the aim of increasing the yield of unreported treatable illness. Barber, Wallis and McKeating (1980) achieved a more selective cohort of patients by using a questionnaire to identify patients in need of screening. Pike (1976) screened only those patients who were currently not on treatment. Each of these methods of selective screening add to the variety of options available and they will be described later. However, clear health benefit has not been demonstrated with these selective methods. It is possible that research is not yet sufficiently sophisticated to achieve this.

By the early 1980s the idea of anticipatory care began to be introduced. This was first described by Van den Dool (1970) in the Netherlands, who, having experienced the workload of formal screening, became aware of the possibility of preventive care being an integral part of normal doctor–patient contact. Stott and Davis (1979) drew attention to the enormous potential of the consultation as an opportunity for preventive care, health promotion and case findings. Similarly, Julian Tudor Hart (1975) has shown the value of the approach when screening for hypertension in his South Wales practice.

GENERAL-PRACTITIONER ATTITUDES TOWARDS SCREENING

An important consideration in anticipatory care is doctor attitude. A measure of this was provided as a result of a postal survey of doctors who were members of the Royal College of General Practitioners in the North West of England (Williams, 1983). A question was included about screening elderly patients. There turned out to be considerable diversity of opinion about its value. Ten per cent of the doctors were already carrying out formal comprehensive screening sessions for elderly patients in their practice. Those who were not doing so were asked whether they would

Table 10.1 Response of non-screening doctors to question of holding screening sessions for elderly people

Response to question	Percentage
Strongly yes	11.5
Possibly	25.7
Don't know	24.8
Doubtful	15.0
Strongly no	23.0

Source: Williams, 1983

be prepared to undertake this type of screening, and to state how strongly they felt about it (see Table 10.1). Only 11% were strongly in favour of screening, and 23% were strongly against. Comments included problems with workload, time and finance. Several doctors pointed out that screening should be financed in the same way as contraceptive care, that is on a fee-for-service basis. Some recognized that there was a need for screening but were unsure of their own commitment to it. Others required to be convinced of the usefulness of screening. When asked which methods they favoured for identifying problems, most preferred to do so during normal consulting time. This is, of course, the basis of anticipatory care. The doctors also stressed the importance of sharing information gathered by other members of the primary-care team, especially health visitors and district nurses.

METHODS AVAILABLE FOR PROVIDING
PREVENTIVE AND ANTICIPATORY CARE

It would appear that no single acceptable method of providing preventive and anticipatory care for elderly people will emerge. Furthermore, it is probably unlikely that in the near future research will come up with a best-buy solution that has proven value. The case for anticipatory care is really made on the grounds of the visible, practical, common-sense benefits derived by individual patients. The time for providing such care is now. The results of sophisticated research to prove health benefit may take up to a decade to produce. To wait for this would mean once again missing the opportunity presented by the growing number of very old persons to provide a good service at a time when it is really needed.

What is available is a menu of preventive-care possibilities that should enable each practice and each primary health-care team to choose the method that satisfies the needs, resources and interests of both the members of the team and the patients themselves. Most of the options are the product of individual enthusiasm and the choice is wide.

The possible methods are: (1) to do nothing except provide the normal service that is available for the rest of the population, (2) to rely on well-

elderly clinics provided by health authorities, (3) to undertake comprehensive screening of total practice populations of over-65s, over-70s or
over-75s, (4) to provide selective screening of, for instance, specific at-risk
groups, (5) to undertake a postal survey of all elderly patients (e.g. over
65 years old), followed by health-visitor or doctor contact if necessary, (7)
to carry out opportunistic case finding at patient-initiated contact and (6) to
organize a health-visitor/nurse, home-visiting, case-finding programme.
Methods four, five and six are systematic case finding exercises; method
seven is an opportunistic case finding exercise. All need to be followed
by a full assessment similar to method three for people found to be in
need of help.

Many community-care teams and practices seek help when determining which type of anticipatory-care programme to initiate and they need
to know about the practical implications of the programme when undertaking the planning. The various methods will therefore be described in
some detail. There are also some interesting local initiatives that are
variations on the major themes and may be relevant in other areas. Some
of these will also be described.

The first two methods on the menu require some comment. The first is
to do nothing. It could be argued that the iceberg of illness is a myth, or at
least minimal. There is evidence that unreported illness is not always
demonstrated and the level may be overstated in the literature. Some
studies in general practice have failed to confirm this amongst their
patients. It is possible that in rural areas, for instance, there are not the
same problems. John Fry (1984), arguing the case against screening, asks
the question 'Checking the elderly – why should we bother?'. He makes
the point that anticipatory care is a normal part of good community care.
This comes close to the parallel argument that in old age things are best
left alone, intervention only upsetting the equilibrium. Added to this, is
the point that the uncritical transfer of findings from the 1960s to the
1980s has led to the exaggeration of under-consultation amongst elderly
people (Ford and Taylor, 1985). The assumption that services must be
provided on a fairly unselective basis for a group who will not take the
initiative themselves is certainly open to question. Recent studies have
cast doubt on the value of an approach which treats elderly people as
having multiple problems until proved otherwise (MacDonald and Rich,
1983). One study (Network for Developmental Initiatives in the Community, 1987) openly rejects professional screening, saying 'Such a
narrowing of perspective (to focus on problems) does little to help older
people reach a level of optimum coping within the limitations of their life
histories and environments'. It is suggested that professionals focusing
on problems deny old people both the recognition of their own individuality and the capacity to control their own lives as far as possible.

There is truth in these arguments, but as Freer (1985) points out, the
overwhelming argument is in favour of an anticipatory approach. As

has been discussed earlier, unreported illness is very often present and although these conditions may be relatively minor, the most important ones already being known to the doctor, they can affect function significantly. An anticipatory programme is therefore helpful and provides an enormous opportunity for a positive approach to healthy living in old age. This is nowadays becoming increasingly accepted as beneficial. However, accepting that there is an argument in favour of continuing to provide normal service, the fact of actually having considered the situation at least alerts the team to difficulties in old age, and it is possible that such review in itself changes practice in many subtle ways.

Some health authorities provide clinics whose objective is to provide check ups for elderly persons. They are usually undertaken by consultants in geriatric medicine and are no doubt very valuable to individual patients. Anything that contributes to healthier living in old age is to be welcomed. These clinics are open access which is in itself good, but unfortunately the patients who are in real need probably never think of attending. A more comprehensive service is needed and this can only be provided through primary care.

REASONS FOR UNDERTAKING ANTICIPATORY CARE

The last four options in the list accept that there is a need for some form of anticipatory care. This is a wide concept involving all types of disease prevention and health promotion. It is convenient at this stage to summarize the reasons for such an exercise.

1. To provide an opportunity to undertake a tertiary-screening or case-finding exercise designed to find unreported medical and social need with the aim of improving functional ability;
2. To identify special at-risk situations where specific follow-up arrangements can be made to maintain regular surveillance;
3. To review existing therapy and make arrangements for appropriate follow-up;
4. To review the social, financial and environmental situation of each old person;
5. To note the functional status of an old person;
6. To alert other organizations (e.g. voluntary organizations) to old persons requiring their help;
7. To inform an old person about the services available in the community, especially those within the practice;
8. To provide health education and advice about self-help, so that the personal autonomy is maintained and enhanced;
9. To update patients' records, e.g. telephone numbers and prime carers;
10. To review any primary preventive needs, e.g. influenza immunization;

11. To review the carer situation;
12. To create a disability register of old people in the practice.

Problems to be solved

Every screening programme has as its aim the solution of a particular problem and this must always be clearly defined. When screening elderly people, the problem is the presence of unreported need. This in turn has three aspects: the presence of unmet need; the vicious-circle effect of several minor unreported conditions leading to reduced functional ability; and why the old person actually did not report need. The solving of these problems is the aim of preventive screening. Finding and treating unreported conditions, especially of a minor nature, is not difficult, but understanding the reasons why old people do not report illness, and at least checking out whether anything can be done to help them, is a deeper consideration. Some of the reasons for non-reporting include inertia, putting symptoms down to old age, a feeling that there is nothing to be done and fear of doctors and institutions. But no work has been undertaken to determine whether an anticipatory service reduces the risk of non-reporting. Hopefully, by educating old persons, such exercises may encourage them to take a positive interest in their own health and to seek help at an early stage. Despite the observations of some commentators there is, however, no evidence that the prevalence of unreported need has changed over the last twenty years and it is possible that the new cohort of elderly people exhibits the same phenomenon as did its predecessor. A reduction in the number of acute medical and social problems may be thought to be possible as a result of anticipatory-care intervention, and this may happen, but a more realistic hope is that when these acute incidents occur, the fact that health workers have better information about patients will allow better management.

Validation

If it is considered that the prime aim of screening is to discover at an early stage established treatable disease that is hitherto unreported, validation is necessary and this has been attempted. It is prudent to be aware of the way in which such validation is undertaken. Many criteria have been used to test whether the stated objectives have been achieved, but a successful screening exercise is usually expected to satisfy the following eight points. For example purposes, the way in which a full comprehensive screening programme might be assessed is included.

1. The screening should be capable of being applied to a specific group in the population and that group should be easily reached.
   Elderly-patient screening is certainly applied to a specific group in the

population. They can be easily identified using a practice age/sex register of old people.

2. The screening process must be clear, easily repeatable, well defined, safe and reliable.

   The procedure is quite clear. Full screening consists of interview and examination, followed by any necessary action. It can be undertaken by either the doctor or the health visitor.

3. It should be practical on a large scale.

   Screening old people is certainly practical in general practice and could be carried out widely. A list of 2200 patients would contain about 125 patients aged over 75. It would take only a year to see these patients at the rate of two per week.

4. It should be cheap.

   The low cost to the community, if it is carried out in general practice, is self-evident.

5. It must be acceptable to patients.

   Most surveys carried out in general practice have shown that the patients accept the procedure and welcome it. The view is often expressed that old patients feel reassured after the full examination as a part of the screen.

6. It must have a satisfactory yield.

   Most studies have shown a high yield of morbid conditions and often the need for social services. The large number of patients needing some type of treatment is frequently commented upon by anyone undertaking this type of work, so the yield expected from this type of clinic can be quite considerable.

7. The conditions isolated at screening should be capable of being effectively treated.

   Unfortunately very few follow-up studies have been done on patients following screening. Lowther, MacLeod and Williamson (1970) evaluated their early diagnostic services for the elderly. They found clear evidence of improvement in half their patients who had carried out the recommendations. If all patients were included, the proportion helped was about 23%. Williams (1974) found similar figures in his followup. Unfortunately, neither reviewed the minor conditions, but experience in practice does seem to indicate that these are very treatable and when this is undertaken, improvement in function is achieved. In the elderly, diagnosis is often needed for prognosis rather than treatment.

8. Does the screening process contribute to the recognition of unreported need and can it be shown to do so by looking at the group studied before and after the exercise?

   Undoubtedly, screening identifies unreported need and both Williams and Lowther found this in their original and follow-up studies. Lowther points out that early detection reduces the period of suffering in many conditions and avoids hospital admission. He states that some merit lies in the mere identification of disease. Unless a diagnosis is made there can be no rational therapy and the questions of prevention can never arise. Whether screening is the answer to the whole problem of unreported need is not clear.

Tulloch and Moore (1979), in a two-year, follow-up programme, found, however, that the screening had made no significant impact on the prevalence of socio-economic, functional and medical disorders affecting health. The study patients were, however, kept independent for longer. There was also a decrease in the expected duration of stay in hospital. Vetter, Jones and Victor (1984), in a study reviewing the effects of health visitors in two practices, showed that the urban health visitor provided significantly more services for the elderly disabled patients and significantly reduced their mortality but not their morbidity. The quality of life was also improved. The rural health visitor, on the other hand, had no such effect. There have also been studies from abroad. Hendrikson, Lund and Stromgard (1984) undertook a three-year, randomized controlled trial in Copenhagen where patients over 75 were given a social and medical assessment by a doctor and visited thereafter at three-monthly intervals. In the study group there was a significant reduction in mortality. The benefits were thought to be due to regular visits and to one person co-ordinating medical and social support. The patients were thought to be better motivated about health and more active and self-confident as a result of this system of care. Another randomized controlled trial carried out in the USA by Rubinstein and his colleagues (1984) involved assessment of patients in a hospital. The study patients had significantly lower mortality, were significantly less likely to have been discharged to a nursing home than their own home and were more likely to have improved functional status than the control group during the study period. There is obviously no clear answer to the question of the effect of screening on health status and the latest studies show that some of the benefits are not easily measurable. This may explain why definitive evidence of health benefit has not been demonstrated and yet it seems clear that there is substantial face-value advantage to be gained.

Dangers

Problems do exist in undertaking formal screening examinations. Enthusiasm is necessary on the part of the doctor and nurse, and there is a risk as a result of overtreatment. The patient's life can be made more difficult by giving too many drugs. It is also possible to make a patient aware of problems which had previously caused no trouble. It would be wrong to upset a patient's equilibrium by unnecessarily drawing attention to these and it might be just as well to note them and say nothing. There may be a danger of medicalizing old age and encouraging people either to expect rapid physical decline on retirement or to relinquish responsibility for self care and independent choice.

But if screening takes place it is vital that negative cases should in fact be negative. It would be disastrous to miss something important and reassure the patient that all was well so that he/she subsequently failed to report symptoms because of this. It is essential that such screening should be through and ongoing.

Another criticism levelled at screening is that the exercise may make the doctor and his team complacent. Once seen, there may be a danger of the old person being forgotten. This is unlikely. If difficulties exist, surveillance is usually instituted. If all is well, guidance will have been given to encourage the patient as to when to report back. It is likely that the patient will be seen during the course of the next few months in the surgery anyway.

Some doctors and members of the primary health care team assert that they already know all their elderly patients and screening is unnecessary. Yet it is surprising how often somebody is examined at a screening clinic who has problems despite having been seen recently by a doctor or having been given repeat prescriptions.

PRAGMATIC ISSUES

Before proceeding to describe in more detail the screening options available, it is necessary to pause and take a wider view of the problem to be solved. As well as a medical literature mainly concerned with how to set up a preventive programme without unacceptably high costs in money and additional workload, there is a sociological literature. This focuses on different perspectives on ageing, particularly dependence and independence. Taking account of these points has led to the general consensus that the problems experienced by the elderly are best approached through the assessment of difficulties with activities of daily living, rather than screening for specific diseases. Help with these difficulties is unlikely to be found solely from doctors and referral to paramedical and social services is likely to be important. An unresolved issue is how broad the assessment should be. It is necessary to formulate clear objectives when considering screening and often pragmatic decisions will have to be made about the extent of the exercise (Perkins, 1988). Furthermore attitudes are important. Health care workers will need to think routinely in terms of function rather than solely of disease. It may be that what doctors do is less important than how they do it (Freer 1987).

In the next two chapters, for completeness, a full comprehensive screening programme and details of the various opportunistic and case finding exercises will be described.

REFERENCES

Barber, J.H. and Wallis, J.B. (1976) Assessment of the elderly in general practice. *J. R. Coll. Gen. Pract.*, **26**, 106–14.

Barber, J.H., Wallis, J.B. and McKeating, E. (1980) A postal screening questionnaire in preventive geriatric care. *J. R. Coll. Gen. Pract.*, **30**, 49–51.

Cowan, N.R. and Anderson, W.F. (1952) Experiences of a consultative health centre for older people. *Public Health*, **74**, 377–82.

Ford, G. and Taylor, R. (1985) The elderly as underconsulters: a critical reappraisal. *J. R. Coll. Gen. Pract.*, **35**, 244–7.

Freer, C.B. (1985) Geriatric screening: a reappraisal of preventive strategies in the care of the elderly. *J. R. Coll. Gen. Pract.*, **35**, 288–90.

Freer, C.B. (1987) Detecting hidden needs in the elderly: screening or casefinding. In *Preventive care of the elderly: a review of current developments.* Taylor, R.C. Bucklay, E.G. (Eds) Occasional Paper 35. Royal College of General Practitioners., London.

Fry, J. (1984) Checking on the elderly – should we bother? *Update*, **29**, 1029–31.

Hart, J.T. (1975) Screening in primary care, in *Screening in General Practice*, Churchill Livingstone, (ed. C.R. Hart) Edinburgh, 17–29.

Hendrikson, C., Lund, E. and Stromgard, E. (1984) Consequences of assessment and intervention among elderly people: a three year randomised controlled trial. *Br. Med. J.*, **289**, 1522–4.

Lowther, C.P., MacLeod, R.D.M. and Williamson, J. (1970) Evaluation of early diagnostic service for the elderly. *Br. Med. J.*, **3**, 275–7.

MacDonald, B. with Rich, C. (1983) *Look me in the eye: old women, ageing and ageism* Women's Press, London.

Network for Developmental Initiatives in the Community (1987) Senior citizens life programme proposals document. University of Bristol.

Perkins, E.R. (1988) *Preventive care of the elderly: a literature review.* Health Education and Promotion Unit, Nottingham Health Authority. (Personal communication).

Pike, L.A. (1976) Screening the elderly in general practice. *J.R. Coll. Gen. Pract*, **26**, 698–703.

Rubinstein, L.Z., Josephson, K.R., Wieland, G.D. *et al.* (1984) Effectiveness of a geriatric evaluation unit. A randomised controlled trial. *New England Journal of Medicine*, **310**, 1664–70.

Stott, N. and Davis, R.H. (1979) The exceptional potential in each primary care consultation. *J. R. Coll. Gen. Pract.*, **29**, 201–5.

Taylor, R., Ford, G. and Barber, H. (1983) *Research Perspectives on Ageing. The Elderly at Risk*, Age Concern, London.

The South-East London Screening Study Group (1977) A controlled trial of multiphasic screening in middle age: results of the South-East London screening study. *Int. J. Epidemiol*, **6**, 357–63.

Tulloch, A.J. and Moore, V. (1979) A randomised controlled trial of geriatric screening and surveillance in general practice. *J. R. Coll. Gen. Pract.*, **29**, 730–3.

Van den Dool, C.W.A. (1970) *Huisarts en Wetenschap*, **13**, 3, 59.

Vetter, N.J., Jones, D.E. and Victor, C.R. (1984) Affect of health visitors working with elderly patients in general practice: a randomised controlled trial. *Br. Med. J.* **288**, 369–72.

Williams, E.I., Bennett, F.M., Nixon, J.V. *et al.* (1972) Socio-medical study of patients over 75 in general practice. *Br. Med. J.*, **2**, 445–8.

Williams, E.I. (1974) A follow-up of geriatric patients: socio-medical assessments. *J. R. Coll. Gen. Pract.*, **24**, 341–6.

Williams, E.I. (1983) The general practitioner and the disabled. *J. R. Coll. Gen. Pract.*, **33**, 296–9.

Williamson, J. (1987) Prevention screening and case finding: an overview, in *Preventive Care of the Elderly: A Review of Current Developments.* (eds R.C. Taylor and E.G. Buckley), Occasional Paper 35 Royal College of General Practitioners, London.

Williamson, J., Stokoe, I.H., Gray, S. *et al.* (1964) Old people at home: their unreported needs. *Lancet*, i, 1117–20.

11   *Organization of a screening programme*

PRELIMINARY WORK

Age/sex register

The first essential is to form an age/sex register for the elderly patients. This can be done with the help of the Family Practitioner Committee for patients aged 65 years and over. Details of the patient's name and address, date of birth, sex and, if known, occupation are included on small cards, which are stored in a standard, metal filing cabinet (the Royal College of General Practitioners provides cards that are suitable for use in an age/sex register). These cards are kept in birthday order, males being separated from females. When the list is first obtained from the Family Practitioner Committee, it is usual to compare details with the practice filing system. Occasionally patients have died or have moved to a new address and the records need updating. An early task is to feed into the system details of patients who are in hospital, welfare homes or nursing homes. These days many practices have their age/sex registers linked to a computer and this has many advantages. Having established the register, the task of keeping it up to date should be given to one member of the practice staff.

Age of entry into screen

There is a difference of opinion as to what is the correct age to start screening. It has been said that the real problem of old age starts around the age of 75 and it is above this age that screening becomes productive. Certainly younger old people retain the ability to report problems. Probably the best age to include patients in a screening exercise is about 72, although this is quite arbitrary and any age between then and 75 would be suitable. An attempt should be made to see all patients over the chosen age. This, in the first place, will need spreading over a couple of years, but once completed, only those reaching the appropriate birthday and those on periodic review will need to be seen.

Who does the screen?
By far the best combination is that of the doctor and the health visitor, with a social worker involved if this is possible. Health visitors may be able to screen old people themselves by asking certain selected questions and looking for important clinical signs. Most significant medical conditions can be found in this way and if need be referred to the doctor. Many of the unreported problems of old people are relatively minor, but nonetheless, full examination is often necessary to discover these. Doctor examination is undoubtedly valuable as it gives the patient confidence, and treatment, referral and investigation can be immediately arranged. Ideally the exercise is one of teamwork involving all members of the practice.

Invitation to the patient
In early screening exercises this was done by letter of invitation explaining the nature of the exercise and asking for co-operation. Enclosed was a prepaid reply card on which the patients were asked if they would co-operate and whether they were able to come to the surgery themselves, whether they needed transport, or whether their condition necessitated a visit from the doctor at home. These early-reply cards worked very well and produced response rates of around 85%, but they could be criticized on several grounds. It was not easy to explain in a letter the exact nature of the screen and the preventive aspects of it. It was difficult for some, particularly very old patients, to understand why the doctor wanted to see them and a few questioned his or her motives. Invitation by letter can also be criticized because of the possibility that a screen could take place without anyone being aware of what the home and environmental circumstances might be. It is therefore sensible to include some kind of assessment of the patient's actual living conditions. For this reason it is probably better if patients are visited by a health visitor and asked if they will participate in the screening exercise. During this invitation visit, an assessment of the housing situation can be made. This method, although more time-consuming, has increased the response of some screens to 100% and has also enabled more realistic transport arrangements to be made. It is, therefore, the method to be recommended.

Transport
This may present certain problems, as transporting patients to general practitioner's surgeries or health centres is not included in the NHS provisions. Sometimes volunteers can be recruited to transport old people to the surgery and it might also be possible for the health visitor or member of the practice staff to undertake the task, providing insurance cover is adequate. In the author's original screening sessions, those people who were unable to make their own way to the surgery were brought by car by volunteers. These car drivers were often recruited from practice patients.

Pro formas

It is useful to have standard check lists for the screen that can be incorporated into the practice notes. These provide a good baseline for any future medical or social incident. The format of a check list does, however, provide problems. The present record system consists of envelopes that are totally inadequate to incorporate any volume of information. Either only a small amount of material is recorded, or an attempt must be made to convert the whole of the over-65 record system into A4 size. There is a lot to be said for reviewing the patient's note system when he reaches his sixty-fifth birthday and converting it to A4. These days, with many practices having computer systems, it may be possible to record the result of the screen on the computer. Another difficulty is to know how detailed to make the assessment of the old person, and hence the check list. Many examples have been produced, but it is probably best for the doctor and health visitor to work out their own schemes. In general, these will be in three sections: the interview, the examination and the final assessment of action and follow-up. A useful guide to questionnaire and examination procedure is given by Milne *et al.* (1972).

THE INTERVIEW

Note on history-taking in old people

There are sometimes difficulties in taking a history from an old person. The memory may be failing, deafness may be present and complaints may not be precise. For these reasons the old patients can fail to give a reasonable account of themselves and when faced with a health visitor or doctor, may still overlook significant symptoms, although some may do better with the health visitor than the doctor. It is therefore useful to have a relative present at a screening clinic, so that information may be confirmed and supplemented. The medical history is often very long and much of it is irrelevant. Considerable discernment is necessary to identify what is important, particularly when the patient is an enthusiastic raconteur. Compared with younger subjects, illness sometimes progresses at different rates in old people and this must be remembered when interpreting symptoms. The fact that a symptom may have been present for some time may not necessarily rule out serious illness. For example, an old person may discount ankle swelling and breathlessness because its development has been insidious. Chronic symptoms may have come to be accepted and disregarded, whereas those that have only just developed within the last few days are given prominence. Different significance is sometimes placed on symptoms by old people; thus, tiredness, which may be due to iron-deficiency anaemia, may be ignored. Some symptoms, on the other hand, such as tinnitus or itching are very distressing and complained of readily. Nevertheless, what is important to the health visitor may not be so to the patient. For these reasons, direct questioning is very necessary to elicit vital information.

General information
Obviously, the name, address, sex, date of birth and marital status need to be recorded, but it is also useful to know the name and address of the next of kin and any relevant telephone numbers. It is also interesting to note when the patient last visited the doctor. Height and weight should also be recorded so that a baseline is available. Past occupations are sometimes relevant.

Social assessment
If a social worker is included in the team, a full professional social assessment may be made. Failing this, it is nevertheless possible and necessary to elicit certain important social information. The idea is to assess the general suitability of the patient's environment and his/her ability to cope with looking after him/herself within it. It is necessary to know whether the patient lives alone, or is housefast, or bedfast. If the old person does live alone, note should be made of how long he/she has done so and what support there is from relatives, friends and neighbours, and how much contact there is with them. If not living alone, the state of health and composition of other members of the household may be relevant. The suitability of the dwelling is also important; it may be a house or flat, rented or owned, and details of the number of rooms and adequacy of the washing, toileting and cooking facilities should be noted. Assessment of heating, ventilation and any possible accident hazards are necessary. The general state of repair of the house should be observed. Functional capacity can be assessed using the Williams' rings model as described in Chapter 14.

Diet
An account of the nutritional state of old people is given in Chapter 13. During the screen it is essential to determine whether an old person is taking an adequate diet. Some direct questions are usually needed and the minimum aim should be for him/her to have one cooked meal per day.

Finance
It is not easy to raise directly the question of financial difficulty. Many people do not receive their full entitlement of allowances, and it may be necessary to give advice about these. Sometimes the person is financially secure but reluctant to spend money on obviously needed items such as clothes, shoes, extra heating and food. Patients occasionally need to be gently persuaded by the health visitor to spend a little of their savings.

Previous medical history
A note may be made of any significant previous illness, injury and operation.

Current medical treatment
The treatment that a patient is receiving at the time of the screen needs tabulating so that it can be reviewed and entered on a co-operation card. It is often interesting to find out if the patient is taking any non-prescribed medication and, if so, what it is.

Problem lists
It is helpful at this stage to draw up a problem list for the patient. This should be divided into non-active problems – these summarize situations that have happened in the past and are no longer a significant consideration, for example, previous anaemia, alcoholism, etc. – and active problems such as bronchitis and osteoarthritis. At this stage it may be worthwhile noting allergies, smoking habits and whether or not the patient is having immunizations.

THE EXAMINATION

The first essential when examining an old person is to make them feel comfortable and relaxed. The room should be warm and the examination couch fixed at such a level that the patient can get on and off easily. The back rest should be at an appropriately high angle, as many old people cannot lie flat. Undressing sometimes presents a problem and the health visitor or practice nurse can help with this. Occasionally an old person will refuse to undress and then it will be necessary to use ingenuity and the 'keyhole' technique where small areas of the body are exposed progressively through gaps in clothing. Many physical changes take place with ageing, and should be taken into account when conducting an examination.

Assessment of general condition
Much can be learned about the patient by merely observing his/her appearance and behaviour. He/she may be clean and smartly dressed or untidy with food-stained clothes, indicating a lack of interest or deteriorating ability for self-care. Watching someone move and climb on to the couch may indicate problems with mobility. The patient's face may display emotions of worry and anxiety or happiness and contentment. How well an old man has shaved or whether an old lady still uses make-up may give a clue as to how much self-interest is retained and also whether good manual dexterity is still present. Speech may show defects such as

slurring or change in pitch. Note should be made of any recent weight loss.

Mental state

General mental alertness and whether the patient is bright and cheerful should be noted. Simple tests such as asking the patient to recall the name of the Prime Minister or more personal facts like his/her own birthday, or home address, can be carried out to determine memory deficiency and inadequate orientation. Early dementias can be recognized in this way. Psychotic illness may also be present and need diagnosing. A knowledge of the patient's previous personality can be helpful in this respect. For instance, if a previously well-dressed man presents a picture of untidiness and lack of personal hygiene, it could indicate the presence of early mental deterioration. Guides to brief assessment of mental state are available (Wilson and Brass, 1973). Useful further tests are given in Keith Thompson's book *The Care of the Elderly in General Practice*, page 251 (Thompson, 1984). A good practical method is the mini-mental state assessment (Folstein, Folstein and McHugh, 1975).

Mobility

Mobility needs assessing on a functional basis, testing, for instance, whether a patient is able to walk, stand, and particularly to do this without loss of balance. Any unsteadiness or restriction of movement can be due to a variety of skeletal and neurological conditions. Examination of both these systems when mobility is being assessed is helpful. Examination of the feet is also important.

Evidence of anaemia

Anaemia is common in old people and routine blood testing is essential, but it is nevertheless interesting, during clinical examination, to make an assessment of the possibility and degree of anaemia. During an examination of nearly 300 patients by the author, an assessment of anaemia was attempted, using as guides the colour of the conjunctiva and the condition of the skin, fingernails and tongue (Williams and Nixon, 1974). The mean haemoglobin level of those showing clinical evidence of anaemia was calculated and compared with the remainder of the group. Evidence of anaemia judged by pallor of the conjunctiva was found to be the best guide, although it must be admitted that it cannot be reliable.

Endocrine system

Most of the endocrine diseases occurring in old age are treatable. Diabetes may be suspected from the history, but it is usually diagnosed by testing urine and blood. Thyroid and adrenal disorders need careful assessment, as there is sometimes a fine line between changes due to old age itself and those due to disease.

Alimentary tract

Examination of the digestive system starts with a look at the teeth. Not all old people are edentate and some have a good set of teeth. These may, however, need treatment and the aim should be to preserve them for as long as possible. Many old people have ill-fitting dentures that they have possessed for many years. Whether these should be replaced rather depends on how the patient is managing. Dental advice is usually necessary. Further examination of the alimentary tract proceeds in the normal way, with a special look at the hernial orifices as hernia is not uncommon.

Possible pitfalls are an enlarged liver, due to distortion of the thoracic cage, a pulsating abdominal aorta, which is often felt in old people and does not necessarily imply an aneurysm, and lumps of hard faeces that are present in the descending colon. Rectal examination also often reveals problems, for instance, haemorrhoids, fistulas and skin lesions. In men, a small, hard prostate may be present and signify neoplasm.

Genitourinary tract

It is important to recognize that overflow incontinence and bladder distension may be present without the patient being aware of it. Gynaecological conditions such as prolapse and vulval abnormality are not uncommon.

Cardiovascular system

A complete examination of the cardiovascular system is necessary as many incipient problems may be found. Interpretation of the findings, however, is often difficult. Wide variations are found in, for instance, blood-pressure levels. If the blood pressure has been taken in both arms and a difference of more than 20 mm Hg is found, it may suggest disease of the intrathoracic arterial system. Arteriosclerosis is often seen and when the arm is bent at the elbow, the so-called locomotor-brachialis sign of the beating radial artery can be observed. Arrhythmias and signs of heart failure should be noted and also the condition of the peripheral pulses, together with the presence or absence of oedema.

Respiratory system

Examination of the respiratory system is along normal lines, remembering the changes in respiratory function in old age. Attention can also be paid to the breasts during examination of the chest with a special watch for any signs of neoplasm.

Eyesight

Visual acuity can be measured by simple functional tests. For instance, an idea of the efficiency of patients' eyesight can be found by asking whether they are able to watch television and read a newspaper, and assessed by seeing if they can read print at a short distance. Visual fields should also be tested and an examination of the fundi, lenses and pupil reflexes undertaken as routine.

Hearing
Hearing can again be measured by simple functional tests such as whether the patient is capable of hearing a shouted or whispered voice. Hearing aids, if worn, should also be tested for their efficiency, and the ears should be examined by auriscope to check for wax.

Skin
The natural changes in the skin due to ageing are discussed elsewhere. Many conditions are, however, often present, which need treatment or point to general disease. Evidence of injury, bruising, ulceration, burns or dermatitis are examples. Signs of vitamin C deficiency can also be detected by examination of the skin and the mucous membranes of the mouth. Rodent ulcers on the face should be noted, and treatment – so successful these days – arranged.

Urine testing
Is it worth testing the urine of patients seen at screening clinics? During the survey undertaken by the author and co-workers in 1972 of patients over 75 years of age (Williams *et al.*, 1972), 272 specimens of urine were examined, of which 6 were found to contain albumen and 10 to contain sugar. Eight of these patients with sugar in the urine were not known to be diabetic and of these 5 resulted in a diagnosis of diabetes mellitus. Most of the patients found to have albumen in their urine were women. One was a man who was found to be suffering from a urinary infection. Assessing the significance of positive findings in the urine is sometimes difficult and usually further investigation is necessary.

Blood tests
It is desirable when screening an old person to undertake a haematological assessment. The possible range of tests is wide. Which to undertake should be made on a common-sense basis and a consultation with a pathologist is necessary to determine which is locally practicable. On a pragmatic basis it may be that haemoglobin, urea and sugar are the investigations that bring most in the way of practical return. However, a full list would probably include:

Haemoglobin
FBC and film
ESR or plasma viscosity

Blood sugar
Blood urea and electrolytes (sodium and potassium)
Chemical profile (calcium, phosphorus, alkaline phosphatase, bilirubin,
  LDH and transaminase)
T_3, T_4 uptake and serum thyroxine
Serum lipids
Serum proteins and possibly electrophoresis
Acid phosphatase
Serum folate and B_{12}

The volume of blood to be taken and the bottles required need to be
arranged with the pathological department, but will usually be in the
region of 20 ml. Fixing of normal parameters will again have to be determined in consultation with the pathologist undertaking the tests.

ASSESSMENT

When the health-visitor interview and the doctor examination are complete, an assessment consultation is necessary to consider the findings
and plan future action. This usually involves the doctor and health visitor
but could also involve a social worker and the community nursing sister.
The assessment has five main parts:

1. to construct a list of the medical and social disabilities found
2. to assess the patient's effective health
3. to prepare action charts and initiate any necessary arrangements and
    treatment
4. to make follow-up arrangements
5. to issue co-operation cards

These will now be discussed in more detail.

Disabilities found
A list of the medical disabilities and social problems need to be compiled.
Some of the diagnoses and problems may perhaps need to be provisional,
pending further investigation and consultation. It is interesting to note
whether the conditions were already known to the practice or whether
they were unreported.

Effective health
In Chapter 3 the concept of effective health was discussed and a definition
given of the main groups. It can be a helpful indicator of the usefulness of
the screen to note whether the effective health of the old person has been
changed as a result of the intervention.

ACTION

The action possibilities (see Table 11.1) are as follows:

1. *Nothing.*   The first possibility is that the patient requires no services, no treatment and no investigation. This occurred in about one-third of the patients in the early surveys undertaken by the author, and this is probably the sort of figure that can be generally expected. The fact that no action is needed does not mean, however, that the patient has not benefited from the screen. Very often during the course of the interview and examination small points are discussed and advice given. These are not necessarily noted as action required. It is possible that most old people receive some general advice. There is also the more subtle benefit that is derived from the patient merely gaining contact with the medical and social services and being reassured that nothing is wrong. It is useful for a patient to be told the correct procedure for contacting the doctor in an emergency and to know how an appointment can be made. A card with the telephone number of the practice can be given. The patient may also be introduced to other members of the practice staff and realize that he/she can have direct access to the health visitor. This is all part of the health-eduction function of the screen.

2. *Note 'at-risk' situations.*   A special note needs to be taken of any problems of diet, finance, accident hazards (including possibility of falls in the house) and difficulties with retirement, work or re-employment. A review of the drugs currently being taken also needs to be made. Special 'at-risk' patients will be recognized at this point.

3. *Treatment.*   Specific treatment often needs to be given for conditions found and perhaps the therapy that the patient is already receiving needs adjustment. The basic principles of drug treatment in old age are outlined in Chapter 16.

4. *Health-visitor surveillance.*   Apart from being involved in the clinic, the health visitor has many other roles to perform when looking after old people. The range of her services is extensive and includes health teaching, direct provision of care and support, follow-up surveillance and liaison with other agencies. She will be interested in social as well

Table 11.1 Action possibilities following geriatric screening: general action list

1. Nothing	8. Nursing services
2. Note of at risk-situations	9. Chiropody
3. Treatment	10. Physiotherapy
4. Health-visitor surveillance	11. Occupational therapy
5. Social services	12. Optician
6. Use of hospital services	13. Dentist
7. Investigation	14. Voluntary services

as medical problems and will be involved in arranging for any necessary social services if a social worker is not available. Follow-up visits may be needed and often discussion with the patient's family. The help of voluntary organizations can be arranged by the health visitor.

5. *Social services.* These are listed in Table 11.2 and discussed more fully in Chapter 9.

6. *Use of hospital services.* Hospital admission may sometimes be necessary for the treatment of some acute condition found at the clinic. This is usually to an acute medical/geriatric ward but may also involve ENT, ophthalmic or psychiatric departments. Admission may be also necessary to geriatric departments for further investigation and particularly for rehabilitation. Occasionally, it might be obvious that an old person is in need of long-stay hospital care. Hospital out-patient referral may be necessary and may involve the full range of specialist care (apart of course from the paediatric and maternity departments!). Domiciliary consultations by hospital consultants are very useful if the patient is housefast or bedfast. Day-hospital care may be appropriate and the advice of the consultant geriatrician is important in assessing this type of case. In some areas there is a half-way-house system, where the GP has access to beds in a general hospital or more usually in a community hospital.

Surgical treatment. The possibilities of surgical treatment in old people have now much improved. It is only in extreme old age that the GP is faced with the problem of whether or not surgery is realistic. Modern techniques now make it feasible to operate on extremely old people in emergencies. Thus, a patient suffering from acute appendicitis or intestinal obstruction should be referred directly to the surgeon. Patients suffering from fractures, particularly of the femur, are treated routinely by plating or hip replacement.

A more difficult problem arises when the patient suffers from a carcinoma in late old age. Whether or not to treat is dependent to some extent on the patient's general condition, but even so, surgical opinion should be sought as palliative measures might become necessary and the surgeon should be involved at an early stage.

7. *Investigation.* A full range of medical investigation is available to old

Table 11.2 Social service possibilities

1. Rehousing	8. Day centre
2. Home help	9. Additional heat
3. Luncheon club	10. Social casework
4. Welfare home	11. Laundry
5. Meals on wheels	12. Appliances
6. Holiday relief	13. Financial aid
7. Blind register	14. Mental-health advice

people and should be used if there is any question of doubt about the diagnosis. Further blood testing, urine analysis and X-rays are easily arranged but more complicated procedures will usually involve referral to hospital consultants.

8. *Nursing services.*   The help of both the practice nurse and the domiciliary nursing team may be needed following screening. The role of nursing care for old people is discussed in Chapter 18.

9. *Chiropody.*   Arrangements can be made for a patient to visit a chiropodist or for treatment to be given at home. This may even be restricted to a simple nail-cutting and foot-hygiene service. Most health authorities have a chiropody service available for old people.

10. *Physiotherapy.*   A full account of the role of physiotherapy is described in Chapter 8. Physiotherapy may be arranged through the hospital or in areas where it exists through domiciliary physiotherapy services.

11. *Occupational therapy.*   Again, this is discussed in Chapter 8. It is usually arranged through the hospital and is particularly suitable for day-hospital care. Some local authorities have occupational-therapy services associated with the provision of aids and appliances. Help is available from them in assessing needs and training in the use of aids.

12. *Optician.*   The services of opticians are no longer available to old people under the NHS. If vision is severely affected, the advice of a consultant opthalmologist is required. Full discussion of these problems takes place in Chapter 19.

13. *Dentist.*   Old people sometimes require dental services either for attention to their own teeth or renewal and adjustment of dentures. Occasionally, it is necessary to arrange for a domiciliary visit to a patient's home.

14. *Voluntary services.*   The help of volunteers is sometimes vital in arranging for the care of old people. Local 'good-neighbour schemes' are to be encouraged and also help with transport, shopping etc. Many organizations exist to help with this type of work and usually the health visitor will be aware of the help available locally.

Follow-up arrangements

Follow up arrangements are important but must be flexible. They are determined by the patient's needs and condition. Sometimes maintenance necessitates continuous supervision, whereas if the patient is in good effective health and not on treatment, there is probably no need for routine examination for maybe three years unless a new situation develops.

Identified at-risk groups need following up at specific intervals, usually by the health visitor or community nursing services. Some patients will have to be reviewed a month after screening to see whether treatment has been carried out and whether services have been provided. This type of review can often be undertaken by the health visitor.

Co-operation card
It is usual at the conclusion of the screen to issue the patient with a card showing the current treatment. This can be carried around by the patient and can then be available to provide information to other doctors and para-medical workers who might be involved subsequently in management.

A CLINIC FOR THE ELDERLY

Out of routine, comprehensive screening of elderly patients came the idea of the organization of a clinic for elderly people. The notion was that such screening should take place at a specific session each week and this should also be the focus of follow-up arrangements. Most patients screened require some sort of action and often need to be seen again. It is also helpful to make some arrangement for review after an appropriate interval. The existence of a specific clinic make it easy to refer patients discovered at case finding for full assessment. A particular situation that can be managed at a clinic for elderly people is discharge from hospital. Co-operation between hospital and community staff in resettlement and rehabilitation can be facilitated. If it is known that such a clinic exists, then hospital workers can make contact with the community or practice staff through it.

REFERENCES

Folstein, M., Folstein, S.E. and McHugh, P.R. 'Mini-mental state': a practical method for grading the cognitive state of patients for the clinician. *J. Psychiat. Res.*, **12**, 189–98.
Milne, J.S., Maule, M.M., Cormack, S. and Williamson, J. (1972) The design and testing of a questionnaire and examination to assess physical and mental health in older people using a staff nurse as the observer. *J. Chron. Dis.*, **25**, 385–405.
Thompson, M.K. (1984) *The Care of the Elderly in General Practice*, Churchill Livingstone, London.
Williams E.I., Bennett, F.M., Nixon, J.V. *et al.* (1972) A socio-medical study of patients over 75 in general practice. *Br. Med. J.*, **2**, 445–8.
Williams, E.I. and Nixon, J.V. (1974) Haemoglobin levels in a group of 75 year old patients in general practice. *Gerontologica Clinica*, **16**, 210–18.
Wilson, L.A. and Brass, W. (1973) Brief assessment of the mental state in geriatric domiciliary practice. The usefulness of the mental status questionnaire. *Age and Ageing*, **2**, 93–101.

12 *Opportunistic and selective case-finding programmes*

OPPORTUNISTIC CASE FINDING

This means case finding that involves expeditious but careful screening during normal contact between patient and health worker. It is consultation-based and to be effective it has to rely on a high proportion of elderly patients having contact during, say, a period of one year with the practice in order to be certain that no-one is slipping through the net. When considering the possibility and feasibility of this type of preventive activity, it was necessary to ascertain what proportion of elderly patients were in fact seen by their doctors regularly.

To do this Williams (1984) undertook a study to investigate what proportion of old people were seen during the course of a year. In two large practices all face-to-face contacts with over-75-year-old patients were recorded. These included home visits by the doctor or deputizing services, surgery consultations, repeat prescriptions and contacts with the district nurse, the health visitor and the practice nurse. The doctors continued their normal practice of clinical care that did not involve any active screening programme although some of the doctors undertook an occasional record review of their patients. Nearly 93% of the population of over-75-year olds were seen in the course of a year. This supports the view that general practitioners see most of their patients reasonably often. This finding was confirmed later by Goldman (1984). Those patients who were not seen during the course of the year were identified and visited by a health visitor. Most of these patients were in good effective health. These findings were also confirmed by Ebrahim, Hedley and Sheldon (1984) studying an over-65 age group. They, together with Williams and Barley (1985), confirmed that these patients were a low-risk group.

It would appear therefore that opportunistic screening of elderly persons, especially those over 75, is a practical possibility. It is therefore necessary to consider how a practice would set about providing this type of care for their elderly patients. Once more, an age/sex register is the starting point. Those over 75 can be identified in the usual way and it is helpful if the records are colour tagged. When undertaking the research described above, it was found to be very easy and helpful to keep a register of attendances and visits of an old person to the practice (see Fig. 16.2, p. 182). This also provides a good method of keeping the age/sex register up to date, but very importantly identifies those who have not been seen. These patients can be visited by a health visitor to test their health and functional status.

It is helpful for the doctor to have a check list as a reminder of important points to consider during a consultation. Each doctor could easily design his/her own, but some guidelines may be helpful. Functional ability is the most important consideration and should be reflected in the list. Possible headings would be mobility, including falls, function of the special senses, brain function, the cardiovascular system, the respiratory system, the gastrointestinal system, the ability to self-care, the identity of carers, drug review and social state. Some of these areas are described in more detail in Chapter 11. Simple tests for mobility, function of special senses, mental state and the various systems can be incorporated into the opportunistic screen. Ability to self-care can also be assessed easily using the principle of the Williams' rings described in Chapter 14. The check list should be relatively short and simple. Health visitors, district nurses and practice nurses should be encouraged to add information to the regular review section in an old person's notes (Russell and Hime, 1988). A good time to start regular review of this type is on the patient's sixty-fifth birthday, when a review of the notes can be undertaken and redundant information discarded. A new problem list and medication list can also be constructed at this time. A check list similar to that produced in Appendix 1 (pp. 265–5) can be made to fit a standard Lloyd George-type envelope. If A4-size notes are used this can be expanded. Alternatively, the results of the screening can be entered into a computer. It is helpful to have available possible action lists and to note what action has been taken. It is very helpful on future occasions to be able to refer back to this so that a check can be made as to whether the action has been undertaken. There is evidence from previous surveys that the referral system is not totally reliable (Williams, in Taylor and Buckley, 1987, p. 38).

This form of case finding is not a one-off exercise. It is part of a continuing process. By having a baseline of health, social and functional status for the patient it is possible by regular review to detect changes and perceive new needs. By doing so, appropriate help can be initiated early and future problems anticipated. At the same time, unnecessary interventions must be avoided and note taken of the wisdom of sometimes leaving well alone, allowing patients to live and manage their own lives.

As Freer (1985) points out, awareness of self-care has increased and the patients have become more involved in the management of their illnesses. It is unrealistic to believe that doctors should bear all the responsibility for the detection of problems in their patients; if changes are to be achieved, patients and their carers must be better informed about health problems and the use of health and other services. Problems can remain hidden simply because the patient thinks it not worth bringing to the doctor and this attitude needs to be diffused by explaining to older people and their relatives how to make the best use of health resources. The better informed the patient, the greater the preventive potential of routine medical care. Freer (1987) has shown in his Southampton practice that opportunistic screening at patient contact is both a feasible and practical activity.

SELECTIVE CASE FINDING

Taylor, Ford and Barber (1983) make the point that most health professionals work on the assumption that some elderly persons are more at risk than others. The risks experienced by such people are special and more likely to be associated with a reduced capacity for self-care and an increased need for various forms of domiciliary care rather than increased susceptibility to specific disease conditions. This possibility of higher levels of need has led to the idea that if anticipatory care exercises are to be more efficient (in terms of yield of unmet need), concentration on those at risk would be beneficial. The most commonly identified at-risk group is probably the very old, that is, those aged over eighty. However, Taylor and his colleagues identified other such groups. They included the recently widowed, the never-married, those living alone, those who are socially isolated, those without children, those in poor economic circumstances, those who have been recently discharged from hospital, those who have recently changed their dwelling, the divorced and separated, those in Social Class V and one important extra group that should be added – those who have no effective prime carer.

   Taylor, Ford and Barber reviewed the nature of the disadvantage experienced by individuals in these groups. They constructed a risk profile for each. This included the strengths and weaknesses in six domains of functioning (health, psychological state, activity, confidence, support and material wellbeing). The most disadvantaged were found to be those recently moved, recently discharged, those divorced and separated and the very old. Taylor, Ford and Barber went on to test the efficiency of these predetermined at-risk groups in selective case finding and concluded that the evidence showed them not to be very efficient. The research also involved a detailed examination of groups based on age, sex and marital status, but disappointingly this also failed to identify an acceptable number of cases. Some pragmatic lessons can, however, be drawn. If the screening is confined to the very old, it is probably worthwhile because there may be increased yield. This fact in itself is helpful to anyone conducting selective screening projects. Similarly, those recently discharged from hospital are worth reviewing. At least some of those who have recently moved house can be easily identified if it has meant a change of doctor. Review at this stage in an old person's life should be helpful. It is necessary, therefore, when considering selective screening, to take account of Taylor, Ford and Barber's work (1983), remembering that special attention to some of those in at-risk situations can turn out to be rewarding.

POSTAL QUESTIONNAIRE

An alternative approach to selective case finding was that of Barber and his colleagues in Glasgow (Barber, Wallis and McKeating, 1980). They have undertaken an extensive research and development programme on geriatric screening, which has depended upon the use of an initial screening letter. The system consists of a method of identifying those who are thought to require a comprehensive assessment. This initial screening is by a short, nine-question postal questionnaire requiring simple 'yes' or 'no' answers. A 'yes' answer to any of the questions or non-reply to the letter indicates that the patient is in need of comprehensive assessment by a practice health visitor. The questions were designed to cover known areas of potential risk to the patient's physical, psychological and social state.

The questionnaire consisted of the following nine questions:

1. Do you live on your own?
2. Are you in a position to have no relative whom you can rely on for help?
3. Do you need regular help with housework or shopping?
4. Are there days when you are unable to prepare a hot meal for yourself?
5. Are you confined to your home through ill health?
6. Is there any difficulty or concern over your health you have still to see about?
7. Do you have any problem with eyes or eyesight?
8. Do you have any difficulty with hearing?
9. Have you been in hospital during the past year?

The screening letter has been shown to be acceptable to elderly people themselves. In Barber *et al.*'s experience (1980) over 80% completed and returned their questionnaire and only 5% refused to have anything to do with it. Both the letter's sensitivity and specificity were satisfactory. Overall, it was assessed as correctly predicting a high proportion of cases. There have been several refinements to these original nine questions. Taylor and Ford (in Taylor and Buckley, 1987, p. 30), for instance, found that four questions (numbers 3, 5, 6 and 8 in the list) succeeded in identifying 83% of all cases at the expense of contacting or visiting 37% of the population of over-60-year olds. Barber (1988) has demonstrated that the use of a letter can reduce the overall workload of a screening initiative by 20%. It is therefore possible that with fewer questions there should be fewer follow-up visits and in turn a further reduction in the total workload. The age range of the patients contacted is clearly critical in these calculations. Undoubtedly the highest yields in terms of unmet need will be in the highest age range. In this method of screening, the health visitor is very involved and the effects on her workload are clearly important. Undoubtedly this type of activity increases the workloads of both the health visitor and district nurse considerably, but possibly decreases the workload of the general practitioner.

The Glasgow system (Barber, Wallis and McKeating, 1980) is flexible and there have been several variations introduced elsewhere. A.W. Cameron and J. Wright (in Taylor and Buckley, 1987, p. 9) in Leeds have used a questionnaire giving more emphasis to the relationship of the patient to the carer. G.I. Carpenter and G.D. Demopoulos (in Taylor and Buckley, 1987, p. 11) in Winchester have used a disability-rating questionnaire, which concentrates very much on functional abilities and activities of daily living. The Edinburgh birthday-card scheme has involved sending each patient in a practice a card on their sixty-fifth, seventieth, eightieth and eighty-fifth birthdays, and including with this a shortened version of the Barber questionnaire (Porter, in Taylor and Buckley, 1987, p. 22). These included:

1. Do you need regular help with housework or shopping?
2. Are you unable to leave your house for any reason?
3. Are there any health problems you have not yet discussed with your doctor?
4. Do you have any difficulty with your hearing that someone is not already helping you with?
5. Do you have someone you can ask to help you if necessary?

This scheme has not yet been fully evaluated, but it demonstrates the type of experiment that is possible. The scheme has had a good response from health visitors and is well received by patients. One 80-year-old wrote back saying 'Thank you for the lovely birthday card – it was the only one I received.'

Most of the development in screening instruments is now taking place in the United States of America. It has become a specialized activity involving a large data set and employing relatively advanced techniques. The Boston ten-item vulnerability index is based on questions that are very functionally orientated and aim to detect the functionally vulnerable (Taylor and Ford, in Taylor and Buckley, 1987, p. 30). The Wisconsin eight-item functional-assessment screen and the Duke University five-item instrumental activities of daily-living screen are similar (Taylor and Ford, in Taylor and Buckley, 1987, p. 30). Most of these instruments use items of daily living in their assessment, but there is variation in how much is included about health status, cognitive function, social support, and income. These instruments very much have a first-stage screening function with a more formal assessment to follow. At present they are used mainly empirically and validation is still only at an early stage. Taylor and Ford (in Taylor and Buckley, 1987, p. 30) in a critical review quote some of the inconsistencies. Screening instruments can be used either to discover hidden need or as an assessment that acts as a filter device prior to entering into a different care system (for example, a nursing home), or for extra-resource allocation. Probably different instruments are needed for these two requirements. The dynamic notion of health and function in old age must be recognized. Many of these instruments can record change over time and a further use may be to monitor these changes within a practice situation.

From the practical point of view a letter on the basis of that used by Barber *et al.* (1980), with possible added questions about availability of carers, would be very useful to individual practices planning screening innovations.

CASE FINDING BY NURSES AND HEALTH VISITORS

The work of Buckley and Runciman (1985) showed that generally, doctors are not good at case finding. Their professional expectations are rarely satisfied by the apparently mundane nature of case finding and they are uneasy about functional assessment. Milne *et al.* (1972) have also shown that nurses could readily detect most of the major afflictions of old age. It is therefore clear that health visitors and nurses are likely to play a very important part in undertaking case finding although as Karen Luker (in Taylor and Buckley, 1987, p. 42) has shown there may be problems associated with fitting work amongst the elderly by health visitors into the remainder of their duties. Nevertheless health visitors are increasingly concerned to get involved with the elderly, in keeping with their professional job definition as family visitors (Goodwin, 1986). Similarly district nurses and paramedical staff are increasingly aware of, and wishing to expand, the preventive side of their work (Lyne, 1984). It has however been calculated that to launch a full screening programme for elderly people throughout the country would require three to six thousand extra health visitors (Barley, 1987), or presumably a similar number of nursing or other paramedical staff. While extra staff may be employed on an *ad hoc* basis by single practices wishing to develop their own programmes, a nationwide screening service could not be staffed without major expansion in the numbers of trained staff or a major reorientation in the workload of those currently employed. Professor James Williamson (in Taylor and Buckley, 1987), analysing the part played by health visitors and nurses, points out that, in the great majority of cases, functional assessment should begin in the patient's home, although the process may be continued in other settings such as health centres. He describes the scope of case finding as being at two levels: first where the nurse observes and acts and second where she observes and refers. The first level concerns assessment by the nurse of any physical, social, mental or family problems that she will deal with herself. The second level concerns physical problems that she identifies and then refers to others for action. Williamson gives a useful check list for undertaking this type of case finding in the Royal College of General Practitioners Occasional Paper 35 (Taylor and Buckley, 1987).

NEW INITIATIVES

As has been described there are two approaches to tertiary screening in elderly people: the universal, which attempts to assess all old people and the selective, which focuses on those most at risk. Examples have already been given of new initiatives associated with the selective method, especially modifications of the postal questionnaire. All these involve a two-stage strategy: firstly to screen out those without obvious problems and then to identify 'cases' amongst the remainder.

An example of new initiatives in comprehensive screening is provided by the Newcastle Care Team for the Elderly Taskforce Scheme (Macleod and Ming in Taylor and Buckley, 1987, p. 19). Here, a team of nurses visits practices to screen all elderly patients. However, a comprehensive exercise can also operate by postal questionnaire as in the Harwich Elderly Assessment Project (Killingback and Sanderson, in Taylor and Buckley, 1987, p. 16). Here, a letter was sent to all patients asking about problems with eyes, ears, teeth and feet, together with some questions about social status. A checkup was also offered and those who accepted were followed up by a health visitor. There was a high response rate to the initial letter and unmet need was demonstrated. In Winchester, trained volunteers have been used to administer a validated questionnaire that formed the basis of a comprehensive screen (Carpenter and Demopoulos, in Taylor and Buckley, 1987, p. 11). In Devon, a trained occupational therapist assessed elderly people in their own homes, again as part of a comprehensive screening scheme (Jones, in Taylor and Buckley, 1987, p. 13). A.J. Tulloch (in Taylor and Buckley, 1987, p. 24) has described an interesting system that he employs in his Bicester practice, which is based on the use of volunteers to collect health-connected data on patients in a systematic fashion, which takes some of the work from the primary health-care team. Clearly there are many opportunities for variations. An approach which takes a more original view of the concept of risk was adopted by Coupland (1986) who followed up elderly people

who had visited the local Accident and Emergency Department immediately after discharge who were not already being visited by their generic
health visitor or district nurse. The study details the needs identified and
action taken, and it seems clear that this sub-group of the elderly has
problems to be tackled.

A recent development which looks like a good solution to the shortage
of professional time and the unsystematic nature of much professional
practice has recently been launched by the Newbourne Group. This
depends on each patient completing and bringing with them at each
consultation a personal health record card. This has been reviewed by
Barber (1988) who found acceptability favourable. However, no evaluation
has taken place and refinement of the record card will no doubt be
necessary.

Approaches to screening from outside the medical framework tend to
stress the individuality of the client and the importance of understanding
his or her own perspective before offering any kind of help. Dant *et al.*
(1987) have developed a biographical approach to assessing the needs of
old people already identified as in need of extra help, which involves
asking the client to talk about the way they have lived their life before
organizing ways in which their current lifestyle should be modified. They
argue that this will reduce the number of inappropriate offers of help
dictated by the professionals' needs rather than the client's and that it is
also in itself a helpful activity, building a client's self esteem.

The Bristol Network Project encourages the setting up of co-operatives
of retired people, members of which seek out and visit old people at risk
with a view to establishing their view of their problems.

Following the publication of the White Paper *Working for Patients* the
Government published a new contract for general practitioners. In it are
detailed services which the GP will be required to provide each year for
patients aged 75 and over. It is stated that the services may be provided
by the general practitioner personally or by a practice team member. The
capitation fee for those patients will be increased. The list is as follows:

1. a home visit at least annually to see the home environment and find
   out whether carers and relatives are available;
2. social assessment (lifestyle, relationships);
3. mobility assessment (walking, sitting, use of aids);
4. mental assessment;
5. assessment of the senses (hearing and vision);
6. assessment of continence;
7. general functional assessment;
8. review of medication.

This amounts to the first part of a case finding exercise. More items need
to be included, but most importantly such an exercise, to be useful, needs

to be followed by a full assessment of patients found to be in need. To do this yearly as part of the general practitioners terms of service marks a major development. The financial and workload implications will need careful consideration. The fact that a social assessment is included is also important as this may herald a change in general practitioner responsibilities in identification and management of social problems amongst the elderly.

OTHER PREVENTIVE MEASURES

Before leaving the topic of preventive measures in old age, it is necessary to consider the value of some office or surgery procedures that are sometimes recommended. These are primary or secondary measures. Many of these are undertaken in younger people, for example, immunization, cervical cytology, mammography, occult blood testing of faeces and routine chest X-rays. The question is often asked as to whether these procedures are of any value in the elderly population.

Immunization

The immunizations that are sometimes advised for an old person are influenza, pneumonia, tetanus and diphtheria. Influenza immunization of elderly patients, particularly those with chronic chest infections, would seem to be sensible and is currently practised in the United Kingdom. Pneumococcal vaccines have been shown to be effective in reducing acute respiratory illness in certain populations, for instance, those discharged from hospital, although they have not been shown to be generally effective in elderly people. Diphtheria immunization is not recommended in the United Kingdom for old people, but it may be useful in other parts of the world. Tetanus vaccination is worth keeping up to date if the old person is involved in an occupation or hobby that involves risk.

Secondary prevention: pre-symptomatic screening

Lung cancer
There is general agreement that chest radiography and sputum cytology to detect lung cancer on a population basis does not have a place in screening elderly people.

Breast cancer
Screening for breast cancer by mammography has proven benefit in all women between 50 and 60 years, but after that it becomes more debatable. It might even be of value up to the age of 65. There is, however, no

evidence that screening of older women by mammography is beneficial. On an individual basis, however, it would seem to be sensible to advise a patient to undertake self-examination well into old age, and during normal care, breast examination should be undertaken.

Cervical cytology
It is generally agreed that cervical smears are not necessary after the age of 65 unless there are existing specific clinical indications, such as previously abnormal smears.

Colonic cancer
There is evidence that searching for faecal occult blood detects pathological colonic tumours at an early stage. There is no evidence, however, that detecting them at this stage actually increases survival rates. Studies are currently being undertaken to find out whether general-practitioner testing for faecal blood increases patients' survival. Until the results of this study are available, it would be premature to undertake these routinely.

Prostatic cancer
It is agreed that plasma acid phosphatase is quite useless as a screening test for prostatic cancer. It is also doubtful whether yearly rectal examinations are indicated, despite the low cost. This is mainly because they are unreliable and much anxiety is generated because of the number of false positives.

Coronary artery disease
Prevention of coronary artery disease in old age is a difficult subject because in a sense damage may already have been done. No-one doubts that the best advice at any age is to stop smoking, to stay normal weight and to remain active. Lipids in elderly people can be ignored; type-2 inherited hypercholesterolaemia cannot be a problem if one has already reached the age of 75. Routine measuring of blood pressure and what to do with a raised level is a problem. There is no really good evidence that diastolic hypertension is a major risk for coronary artery disease in the 65-and-over age group. Nevertheless really high blood pressure and target-organ failure should be looked for. This, however, means measuring many blood pressures and treating only a few. The blood-pressure levels at which treatment is indicated are still uncertain. The risk of cardiovascular disease increases with blood pressure at all ages and in both sexes. However, treating raised blood pressure in elderly persons is not without risk from unwanted effects of drugs and from interactions with drugs taken for other diseases. Clinical studies, including the European Working Party on High Blood Pressure in the Elderly (Amery *et al.*, 1985)

and Coope and Warrender's (1986) randomized trial of treatment of hypertension in elderly patients in primary care, have not really given a definitive answer as far as cardiac mortality is concerned. It is probable that patients over 75 should not be treated for a raised blood pressure and those under this age should only be considered if the blood pressure is over 160 mm Hg systolic and/or 105 mm Hg diastolic. The decision, however, often depends upon the patient's ability to comply, side effects, for instance postural hypotension, and the presence of other diseases.

Stroke

Similarly, there is evidence from the aforementioned studies that treating young old people for hypertension reduces the incidence of stroke, although it might only be marginal. The position regarding the older old is still very equivocal. Prevention of stroke in old age is probably best done by treating hypertension in middle age or earlier. Sometimes in old age the hazards of treatment are greater than the possible benefits.

Although epidemiological evidence that many of these procedures are beneficial is absent, nevertheless when dealing with an individual patient at routine assessment it may well be that some of them could be helpful. General counselling about smoking, weight, alcohol, exercise, accident avoidance and safe driving is probably the most effective measure.

REFERENCES

Amery, A., Birkenhager, W., Brixko, P., Bulpitt, C. *et al.* (1985) Mortality and morbidity results from the European Working Party on High Blood Pressure in the Elderly trial. *Lancet*, **i**, 1349.

Barber, J.H. (1988) Self screening by the elderly using a new personal health record. *Health Visitor*, **61**, 73–4.

Barber, J.H., Wallis, J.B. and McKeating, E. (1980) A postal screening questionnaire in preventive geriatric care. *J.R. Coll. Gen. Pract.*, **30**, 49–51.

Barley, S. (1987) An uncompromising report on health visiting for the elderly. *Br. Med. J.*, **194**, 595–6.

Buckley, E.G. and Runciman, P.R. (1985) Health Assessment of the Elderly at Home. Research Report, University of Edinburgh Library.

Coope, J. and Warrender, T.S. (1986) Randomised trial of treatment of hypertension of elderly patients in primary care. *Br. Med. J.*, **293**, 1145.

Coupland, R. (1986) Effective health visiting for elderly people. *Health Visitor*, **59**, 299–300.

Dant, T., Carley, M., Gearing, B. and Johnson, M. (1987) Identifying, assessing and monitoring the needs of elderly people at home. Care of elderly people at home. Project paper 2. Open University and Policy Studies Institute.

Ebrahim, S., Hedley, R. and Sheldon, M. (1984) Low levels of ill health among elderly non-consulters in general practice. *Br. Med. J.*, **289**, 1273–5.

Freer, C.B. (1985) Care of the elderly. Old myths. *Lancet*, **ii**, 268–9.

Freer, C.B. (1987) Consultation-based screening of the elderly in general practice:

a pilot study. *J. R. Coll. Gen. Pract.*, **37**, 455–6.

Goldman, L. (1984) Characteristics of patients aged over 75 not seen for one year in general practice. *Br. Med. J.* (letter), **288**, 645.

Goodwin, S. (1986) Health visiting for the health of the aged. *Health Visitor*, **59**, 319.

Lyne, P. (1984) 'Just repairing the damage?' Health education and the professions allied to medicine. Health Education Council, London.

Milne, J.S., Maule, M.M., Cormack, S. *et al.* (1972) The design and testing of a questionnaire and examination to assess physical and mental health in older people using a staff nurse as an observer. *J. Chronic. Dis.*, **25**, 385–405.

Russell, F. and Hime, M. (1988) Functional screening of elderly people living at home. *The Practitioner*, **232**, 889–92.

Taylor, R.C. and Buckley, E.G. (eds) (1987) Preventive care of the elderly: a review of current developments. Royal College of General Practitioners, London, Occasional Paper no. 35, March.

Taylor, R.C., Ford, G. and Barber, H. (1983) Research perspectives on ageing. 6. The elderly at risk. Age Concern Research Unit.

Williams, E.I. (1984) Characteristics of patients over 85 not seen during one year in general practice. *Br. Med. J.*, **288**, 119–21.

Williams, E.S. and Barley, M.H. (1985) Old people not known to the general practitioners: low risk group. *Br. Med. J.*, **291**, 251–4.

13 *Nutrition and hypothermia*

NUTRITION IN THE ELDERLY

Both doctors and social workers may be interested in the nutritional state of old people, and it is sometimes necessary to assess whether they are getting adequate nourishment and to advise on proper food intake. This is particularly true of those who may be too apathetic to cook proper meals, such as the very old, those living alone and the disabled. It is useful, therefore, to have some idea of how to assess a person's nutritional level and to understand the causes of poor food intake so that they may be identified and avoided.

It is not easy to be dogmatic about the ideal level of nutrition and there are considerable differences in the needs of people in general for energy and nutrients. These variations persist into old age. Body size, sex and physical activity are all factors that influence need. The quality of the food and the ease with which it is absorbed are also relevant. However, with increasing age, there is a gradual decrease in physical activity and a decline in metabolism at rest. It is to be expected, therefore, that the food intake of old people will be reduced and this ideally should be evenly distributed throughout the diet. Under these circumstances, where there is a balanced reduction of the various foods, malnutrition should not occur. This is probably true for most elderly people, but there are circumstances where faulty nutrition may be present.

How prevalent is malnutrition? Early surveys tended to find a fair amount of inadequate food intake and established cases of vitamin C deficiency were sometimes encountered. Many of these studies were on patients admitted to hospital and perhaps were not typical of the elderly population in the community. Early studies, such as those of Exton-Smith and Stanton (1965), found that although food intake decreases with advancing age, many of the elderly subjects managed to eat a varied diet. A nutritional survey of elderly people carried out by the DHSS (1972) found some overt malnutrition, but not much; the report stresses, however, that many are vulnerable and the margin of safety may be slight. There is obviously the need to identify and treat individuals at risk so that malnutrition may be avoided.

Clinical assessment of nutrition

Assessment of the nutritional status of an old person is therefore important but can be difficult. It is necessary for a doctor or health visitor to find out whether a person is getting enough food and the methods available for doing this are often unreliable and vague. Under these circumstances, it is necessary to rely on physical examination to determine whether the patient is well nourished. This may also present difficulties as specific signs of malnutrition may be totally lacking. Weight loss is an important feature but examples of serious undernutrition with severe weight loss are rarely encountered apart from in some cases of senile dementia. More moderate weight loss may be due to undernutrition, but interpretation is difficult as it may be due to several other causes. Ageing itself results in reduction in body mass and concomitant disease can also influence weight.

Clinically, poor nutrition can show itself in general apathy and lassitude. Unexplained anaemia may well point to an inadequate diet. Some of the factors likely to lead to subnutrition may be present and these will be discussed shortly. Reduction in subcutaneous fat and skinfold thickness is sometimes regarded as a sign of poor nutrition. There may also be, apart from reduction in calorie and protein intake, an inadequate supply of vitamins in the diet and there is evidence to suggest that this can occur in up to half the elderly population. Although the lack of one vitamin, such as vitamin C, may occur in isolation, the signs of frank deficiency and disease are usually due to several different food factors being absent. When assessing the nutritional status, it is therefore essential to take note of any possible vitamin deficiency. Old men living alone may sometimes show signs of vitamin C deficiency; small haemorrhages may be the only sign and these may be seen particularly in the gums and under the tongue. Confirmation can be obtained by assessing the level of ascorbic acid within the white blood cells and platelets. Early diagnosis of osteomalacia caused by vitamin D deficiency should be made biochemically since, when X-ray changes have occurred, the situation is often too late.

Factors affecting nutrition

Physical changes occur in old age that can contribute to a reduction in food intake. The teeth, for instance, are often lost and although chewing is possible without them, it becomes more difficult. Dentures may be unsatisfactory and might limit the choice of foods. Loss of taste and smell can reduce the appetite in old people. The flow of saliva also decreases as age advances, and this may make chewing more difficult. Oesophageal and gastric mobility may be impaired and gastric secretion reduced. This may affect food absorption as also may the presence of a previous partial gastrectomy.

General physical debility is an important cause of undernutrition. The presence of such diseases as heart failure, chronic infection and arthritis can decrease an old person's interest in food. Some drugs may interfere with the absorption of certain vitamins, notably folic acid. These include phenytoin, phenylbutazone and nitrofurantoin. The mental state of an old person may also influence dietary intake. It is likely to be reduced in patients with depression or early dementia. Sometimes dietary fads persist and are exaggerated in old age. A gastric diet may be maintained for far longer than is necessary and may actually contribute to undernutrition. On the other hand, diet may be well maintained despite quite severe behaviour disorder. Alcoholism may be present and may be responsible for a loss of appetite, a fact that is often hidden from the doctor and relatives.

Various environmental factors can influence the food intake of old people. The actual physical preparation of food may be difficult. Kitchen layouts and cooking facilities may be unsuitable for the frail and disabled. Regular shopping for fresh supplies may not be undertaken because of reduced mobility. The author assessed the diet of 207 over-75-year-old people (Williams *et al.*, 1972). One cooked meal per day was considered to be the lowest acceptable level of food intake and 28 were found to be below this. The numbers were relatively small, but it was found that inadequate diet was commonest in Social Classes IV and V and amongst women aged between 80 and 90 years. Those living alone were also more likely to be poorly fed. It was found that the effective health of those on a poor diet was often diminished and also, as an interesting footnote, that the mean haemoglobin level of patients on an inadequate diet was less than the group as a whole. These patients were not clinically malnourished but were obviously very vulnerable. How much was cause and effect is difficult to determine; perhaps once more, a vicious circle is established where patients in poor health or with a low haemoglobin level become apathetic about food and reduced nutritional intake makes the condition worse.

Nutritional requirements in old age

The Department of Health and Social Security has published a booklet on recommended daily amounts of nutrients for population groups in the United Kingdom. The levels suggested for elderly people are given in Table 13.1. Not all commentators agree with these recommendations and they are not necessarily minimal requirements; nor are they much help in determining nutritional status, as lower levels may still be compatible with good health. It must be also remembered that they relate to population groups or subgroups and that the needs of individuals can vary in health as in disease. Nevertheless, they are a reasonable guide and may

Table 13.1 Recommended daily amounts of food energy and some nutrients for population groups in the United Kingdom (assuming a sedentary life)

Age range (years)	Energy (MJ)	Energy (kcal)	Protein (g)	Thiamin (mg)	Riboflavin (mg)	Nicotinic acid equivalents (mg)	Ascorbic acid (mg)	Vitamin A retinol equivalents (µg)	Calcium (mg)	Iron (mg)
Men										
65–74	10.0	2400	60	1.0	1.6	18	30	750	500	10
75+	9.0	2150	54	0.9	1.6	18	30	750	500	10
Women										
55–74	8.0	1900	47	0.8	1.3	15	30	750	500	10
75+	7.0	1680	42	0.7	1.3	15	30	750	500	10

Source: Committee on Medical Aspects of Food Policy (1979)

be useful in planning diets for old people. The current intake of fat in the United Kingdom represents over 40% of the energy consumed. The National Advisory Committee on Nutritional Education (NACNE) (1983) has recommended that in the short term fat should be reduced to 34% of energy and in the long term to 30% of energy. The Committee on Medical Aspects of Food Policy (COMA) report on diet and cardiovascular disease (DHSS, 1984) recommended that 35% of food energy be derived from total fat. All these figures are practical on the assumption that the energy intake is adequate for the individual and that the individual has a good appetite. If an elderly person has a poor appetite, the first essential is to ensure adequate energy intake. This may result in the need to give the same energy in smaller bulk and this would mean more fat and less complex carbohydrate. The need to prevent the risk factors associated with coronary heart disease, which would include a high fat intake, may take second place when considering an elderly person's need for an adequate calorie intake to maintain body weight and body temperature. Adequate fibre in the diet is also now thought to be important.

Nutritional help for the elderly

Good dietary habits should start at an early age, and hopefully these will be continued into advanced years. Accepting that inadequate diet is a possibility, its early detection is important. It can easily be overlooked and it is necessary for doctors, health visitors and social workers to be constantly alert to the possibility. Certain groups already mentioned are vulnerable and need special attention. Opportunistic screening is helpful in recognizing those at risk. Making sure that old people have adequate dentures can reduce subnutrition and anaemia. Those who provide meals on wheels and supervise luncheon clubs can also recognize those whose appetites are poor or whose interest in food is deteriorating. Home helps are also valuable in helping old people to receive adequate nutrition. General education in the principles of nutrition should be part of the primary health-care-team's role, particularly in advocating the necessity to eat fresh fruit or fruit juice and food rich in vitamins A and D, such as oily fish. Advances in technology have meant better packaging of food and much of it now is easy to prepare.

Refrigerators and freezers have meant that storage is now possible for much longer periods and this may be invaluable when patients are incapacitated for a short period. Unfortunately, some old age pensioners do not have these facilities. The wisdom of adding extra vitamins to the diet either as pills or by fortifying foodstuffs is debatable. Excess of vitamins A and D, for instance, can be a hazard and in general, with a well-balanced diet, additional vitamins should be unnecessary, except perhaps in winter for the housebound.

Old people with low incomes tend to buy cheaper foods and sometimes there is the dilemma of priorities as to whether money should be spent on other essentials such as fuel and clothing. Pensioners with special dietary needs are advised to seek Income Relief and should consult social-security officers. To overcome any unsuitable domestic arrangements for cooking, it is sometimes helpful for social workers to advise on alterations and special utensils. Easy access to ovens, shelves and storage units can enable a disabled person to cook, when previously this was proving difficult. Teaching an old person to use these facilities is usually necessary. Meals on wheels and luncheon clubs are, of course, very important and great care is usually given to their nutritional content. Those living alone should be encouraged to use these facilities, especially if they can arrange to eat with others, as this is often a stimulus to the appetite. Finally, there is the problem of obesity which, like in other age groups occurs also in old age. This often shortens life expectancy and can aggravate many other problems. Help from hospital or community dieticians is often necessary to construct suitable diets.

HYPOTHERMIA

By definition, hypothermia is said to occur when the temperature of the body core (that is, deep internal temperature) is less than 35°C (95°F). The condition was first described by Helen Duguid and her colleagues in 1961. Of the 23 cases she described in her Scottish study (Duguid, Simpson and Stowers, 1962), 22 were elderly people. The Royal College of Physicians (1966), in a study involving ten British hospitals, found a temperature of less than 35°C in 0.68% of admissions. Although it is perhaps dangerous to extrapolate from these figures, it could be that several thousand people are admitted to hospital each year with a diagnosis of hypothermia. What the true incidence of the condition is in the community must at the moment be unknown, but it is probable that in winter it is not uncommon. Between four and five hundred deaths annually in Britain are said to be due to hypothermia, but this is probably a low estimate because the illness is not necessarily recognized or included in a death certificate.

Temperature

There are two aspects of body temperature. There is deep temperature, sometimes known as core temperature, around the vital organs, which is maintained constantly despite variations in external conditions. Also, there is the temperature of skin and subcutaneous tissues, sometimes described as shell temperature, which varies with external temperature. In elderly people, deep body temperature is about half a degree lower than in young people and this difference tends to increase as age advances.

Accurate recording of temperature is important when the possibility of hypothermia is present. Most clinical thermometers have as their lower reading, 35°C. Special thermometers are therefore necessary to record low temperatures in old people. Care is needed to shake down the level of mercury sufficiently, for if this is not done the temperature of the body may be lower than the actual reading. The usual method of oral measurement gives only shell temperature. For assessment of core temperature, rectal measurement is necessary. Sometimes this is inconvenient, and some surveys have overcome this difficulty by measuring the temperature of the urine immediately after it has been passed. This is, however, outside the scope of normal clinical practice.

Heat regulation

Maintenance of body temperature involves a fine balance between heat gain and heat loss. Physiologically, a point is set within the body that indicates the temperature required and any difference is registered in the hypothalamus, which sets off appropriate mechanisms for heat loss or gain. Peripheral cold reactors are stimulated when the body is exposed to cold and alternatively, when overheating is the problem (as for instance when pyrogens are released during infections), the hypothalamus is stimulated to activate heat-controlling mechanisms. Many factors affect these delicate mechanisms and an important one as far as elderly people are concerned is the relationship of mass to body surface. An animal with a large body mass, but a small body surface area, will have more difficulty in losing heat and special mechanisms will have to be introduced to allow this to happen. A thin, wasted old person on the other hand, with a large body surface, may have difficulty in conserving body heat and this may sometimes prove to be impossible. This may account partially for the impairment of temperature control that is seen in some old people. The hypothalamus has a higher threshold of sensitivity in the old. Also they cannot respond to hypothalamic stimuli, e.g. by shivering.

Causes of hypothermia

Although hypothermia is principally a condition of old age, it can also be found in babies and infants. Young people, such as climbers, potholers and yachtsmen who find themselves exposed for long periods to cold, wet conditions, can also suffer from hypothermia. The real cause is exposure to cold, but there are factors that exaggerate the effect of this. Impaired physiological maintenance of body temperature seems to be present in some people and this may make them more vulnerable. Many illnesses may be associated with impaired thermoregulatory mechanisms, for instance myxoedema, hypopituitarism, diabetes, stroke, myocardial infarctions, infections and extensive skin lesions. Immobility produced by conditions such as arthritis, Parkinsonism and mental impairment can also be associated with hypothermia. Certain drugs, such as chlorpromazine (Largactil), diazepam (Valium) and, of course, alcohol can also be contributory. This is important when dealing with confused old people because sometimes the confusion may be due to hypothermia, and the use of phenothiazone tranquillizers (e.g. Largactil) may aggravate the hypothermic condition. The environment is also important. People living in cold draughty houses, particularly those in high or exposed conditions, may be particularly vulnerable.

Clinical manifestations

In an established case of hypothermia, the patient is obviously cold and this applies particularly to the abdomen and trunk. Strangely enough, he or she may not complain of cold. Other appearances have been described and include skin of a pale or pinkish colour, which is sometimes puffy and has a resemblance to myxoedema. The voice may also have a deeper tone than normal. The muscles may be rigid and the reflexes sluggish. Consciousness may be clouded and the patient may be drowsy. The pulse is usually slow and the blood pressure reduced. Breathing may be shallow and there may be signs of bronchopneumonia, although hypothermia can mask this condition, and it is only when the patient is warmed that it becomes apparent. A situation seen in the community that is associated with hypothermia is where the old person has for some reason fallen out of bed. There may also be a fracture, particularly of the femur. The patient is usually unable to get back into bed and lies all night scantily clad in a cold bedroom. Discovery may not be for several hours and this type of exposure can lead rapidly to hypothermia. Hypothermia developing insidiously in old people is also very common and much more difficult to identify.

Treatment

It is possible to treat mild cases of hypothermia at home providing that there is adequate care available and that the social conditions in the house are reasonable. The basic principle of treatment is slow rewarming and this is done best by nursing the patient in bed at a room temperature of about 25°C (70°F) so that deep body temperature can be allowed to rise gradually. This means insulating the whole body, especially the head, and giving warm drinks to raise the temperature of the core. Other methods such as rapid rewarming by immersion in a warm bath, although effective in young people, are not to be recommended when dealing with old patients. The vasodilation caused by this quick surface heating may lead to a drop in core temperature and to disastrous circulatory collapse. The disadvantages of the slow method of rewarming the patient are that the hypothermia is prolonged and irreversible changes in the tissues may take place. With mild hypothermia, this is, however, unlikely. Other cases should be admitted to hospital where, although conservative treatment is still indicated, precautions such as barrier nursing, isolation and broad-spectrum antibiotic therapy can be instituted. Severe hypothermia demands specialist treatment and often admission to an intensive-care unit. The outlook for patients suffering from severe hypothermia is not very good. Where the initial temperature is below 30°C, mortality is high.

Prevention

Hypothermia is basically preventable. Colder countries, such as Sweden, do not experience the condition. Economic factors in the United Kingdom are clearly important in contributing to low domestic temperatures in the houses of old people. Elderly people should live in warm surroundings and this should include not only downstairs rooms but also bedrooms. The ideal temperature is between 65°F and 70°F or about 21°C. The cost of fuel is often a problem. Central heating, of course, is ideal, particularly when it is automatic. Electric heating is also satisfactory but expensive. The work associated with coal fires and the danger of paraffin heaters make these two fuels unsuitable for old people. Windows should be closed at night and special attention should be paid to insulation. Double glazing, draught exclusion and roof insulation not only help to reduce the size of the fuel bill but add greatly to comfort. If it is impossible to heat the whole house it is better in the winter for the old person to live in one room and bring the bed down to the sitting room, which can then be kept at a reasonable temperature. People should be well clothed in bed; night-caps and bed socks are recommended. Electric blankets are useful, but may be dangerous if the patient is incontinent. Specially waterproofed electric blankets and low-voltage overblankets, which use very little electricity and are safe, are now available.

Medical and social workers should be alert to the possibility of hypothermia and be aware of the people especially at risk. This could include all those over 75 and those living alone. There seems to be a certain section of the elderly community who have an idiopathic reduction in the body-temperature stabilizing mechanism. The problem is recognizing these people. Perhaps wider use of the low-reading thermometer might help. Doctors should always be alert to the possibility of hypothermia and be careful in prescribing drugs, particularly tranquillizers, to those at risk.

REFERENCES

DHSS (1972) Panel of Nutrition of the Elderly. *DHSS Report on Health and Social Subjects, no. 3: Nutritional Survey for the Elderly*, HMSO, London.

DHSS (1979) Committee on Medical Aspects of Food Policy *DHSS Report on Health and Social Subjects, no. 15: Recommended daily amounts of food energy and nutrients for groups of people in the UK*, HMSO, London.

DHSS (1984) Committee on Medical Aspects of Food Policy *DHSS Report on Health and Social Subjects, no. 28: Diet and Cardiovascular Disease – Report of the Panel on Diet in relation to Cardiovascular Disease*, HMSO, London.

Duguid, H., Simpson, R.G. and Stowers, J.M. (1962) Accidental hypothermia. *Lancet* **ii**, 1213.

Exton-Smith, A.N. and Stanton, B.R. (1965) *Report of investigation into the diets of elderly women living alone*, King Edward Hospital Fund, London.

National Advisory Committee on Nutrition Education (NACNE) (1983) *A discussion paper on proposals for nutritional guidelines for health education in Britain*, Health Education Council, London.

Royal College of Physicians (1966) *Report of Committee on Accidental Hypothermia (1966)*, Royal College of Physicians, London.

Williams, E.I., Bennet, F.M., Nixon, J.V. *et al.* (1972) Socio medical survey of patients over 75 in general practice. *Br. Med. J.*, **2**, 445–8.

14   *Assessment*

For nearly twenty years the subject of assessment of elderly persons, both medically and socially, has lacked clarity. There has been confusion as to the purpose of such assessment, when and by whom it should be undertaken and what it should include. In 1987 a working group on multidisciplinary health assessment of elderly people sponsored by the Kellogg Foundation and supported by the WHO met in Gothenburg, Sweden, to consider some of these issues. The result is a report that gives clear answers to most of the questions raised and by focusing on some difficulties points to areas that need further research. The opening chapter of the report by John Brocklehurst and Franklyn Williams summarizes the group's findings. It gives an excellent and concise account of the place of assessment and with the authors' permission it is used as the basis of this section.

Assessment means the detailed investigation of an individual's total situation in terms of physical and psychological state, functional status, formal and informal social supporters and the physical environment. The need for assessment of elderly persons arises principally from actual or potential breakdown of independent living. Breakdown in old age is complex and must be seen as a failure of equilibrium, often brittle, in which the effects of biological ageing, multiple pathology, harmful effects of drugs and social vulnerability are balanced against a person's physical and mental health. Family and neighbour support, help from statutory or voluntary services, and the commonly overlooked desire of people to retain their independence also enter the equation. Because of this complexity, assessment needs to be comprehensive and several disciplines need to work closely together as a team. When problems have been identified and needs assessed, it is possible to plan subsequent provision of support, rehabilitation or resettlement. To do this sensibly, information must be shared between the various professionals involved. The purpose of assessment is therefore to determine the needs of the elderly person and carers, including the needs that are met and those that are unmet. Thereafter, a programme is evolved and implemented in a way that meets these needs.

WHEN IS ASSESSMENT INDICATED?

The Kellogg Working Party (1987) suggested that multidisciplinary assessment of elderly people should be undertaken for four main reasons: (1) to prevent breakdown (2) to deal with incipient breakdown (3) to deal with actual breakdown (4) on an occasional basis to monitor long-term care. These will now be discussed in more detail.

Preventive assessment

This is mainly undertaken within the framework of primary care and the details of comprehensive assessment are given in Chapter 11. The primary-care team is well developed in a number of countries (for instance, in many health-centre-based general practices in the United Kingdom), but may be absent in others where the first medical contact is with a physician unsupported by a community nurse or social worker. Although it is possible for a comprehensive medico-social assessment to be undertaken in primary care as part of a preventive screening programme, in practice this does not happen very frequently. More commonly, preventive assessment follows anticipatory or opportunistic intervention or a case-finding programme. Both of these have been discussed fully in Chapter 12. Opportunistic screening depends upon the fact that 90% of over-75-year-old patients are seen at least once within a year by their primary-care physician, and the majority of those who are not seen are in good health. The opportunity arises, therefore, for the physician, having dealt with the presenting problem, to carry out a brief screening procedure to include physical function, mental status and social need, and so to identify incipient problems. Case finding usually by other health workers means identification of individuals who are experiencing medical or social prolems. Whichever identification method is used these patients need to be referred for full assessment.

 Case finding should primarily concentrate on old people at risk, probably those recently discharged from hospital, recently bereaved, recently relocated, those suffering from chronic disabling conditions or those requiring repeat prescriptions. The most suitable person to carry out stage case finding is probably the health visitor (public health nurse); however it may be undertaken by the physician or other member of the team. The important point about preventive assessment is that the initiative comes from the professional. In general, the assessment is part of the service offered to old people within primary care. It usually takes place in a doctor's office or surgery, but occasionally also in the patient's home.

Assessment at incipient breakdown

When breakdown is threatened, advice is likely to be sought by the old person or carers. The form in which the assessment takes place varies between countries, but it is always multidisciplinary. In the UK it can take place in the patient's home, in the nursing or welfare home or occasionally, at a health centre. But it may also take place as in other countries in an out-patient, geriatric assessment unit. In the UK this usually follows referral of the patient by a primary-care physician or social worker. Occasionally, an assessment may take place in a geriatric day centre or day hospital. In some countries, for example, Canada, assessment is available through an independent community office that responds to all such enquiries by elderly persons facing breakdown or from their carers and relatives. It is staffed by a nurse and social worker who make a preliminary contact with the old person in his/her own home, making as full assessment as they can and referring for further advice (medical, psychiatric and functional) as they think appropriate. When assessment is complete, these findings are presented to a larger panel representing appropriate disciplines and decisions are taken by this panel about further assistance.

Assessment at actual breakdown

When breakdown occurs, assessments may occasionally be carried out on an out-patient basis, but more often hospital admission will be required and this should be to a geriatric assessment unit. Admission may be directly from home either following an initial domiciliary visit by the consultant or at the request of a primary-care physician. It may also be through accident and emergency or it may be by transfer of the old person from other hospital departments after the precipitating acute problem has been dealt with. In any case this in-patient assessment consists of a nursing, medical, social and functional assessment with further information being obtained from other specialists as indicated. It will involve medical treatment and rehabilitation. The old person's situation and future are usually considered at one or more multidisciplinary case conferences prior to discharge, either to their own home or to some other more appropriate location.

Periodic assessment in long-term care

While episodic medical care is available to all patients in nursing homes and long-stay hospitals, it is necessary also that periodic multidisciplinary assessment should be carried out, and this should involve the nurse, the physician, the social worker and probably the therapist as well. Such a review should assess whether the placement remains appropriate and should consider medications, state of continence, social visits and recreational activities. Similarly, in primary care, periodic review is also necessary following initial preventive assessments. These can be carried out as part of an anticipatory-care programme during doctor – patient contact or by built-in assessments on a regular basis for individuals who are in especially at-risk categories.

THE CONTENT OF MULTIDISCIPLINARY ASSESSMENT

The typical situation calling for assessment is a frail old person facing a serious threat to continued independent living due to complex interactions. This may be physical deterioration, but very often there is also mental decline and increasing inability to perform adequately in the home. Assessment must be inclusive of all the important contributory elements. The following list summarizes such an assessment.

1. A complete medical check-up including history, physical examination and appropriate laboratory studies. Specific attention to status of vision, hearing, dentition, nutrition and medications, including information on accuracy of medication-taking.
2. Mental assessment including objective measures of memory and cognition, mood/affect, evidence of alcohol or drug addiction.
3. A functional assessment, which should include both actual performance as well as ability to perform personal activities of daily living and domestic daily activities.
4. Social history and social status should be examined, including the support network available, primary as well as secondary carers and evidence of emotional as well as physical support, financial status, coping ability and formal and informal services already being used.
5. Environmental assessment including housing conditions, heating, cleanliness, telephone, safety hazards, neighbourhood suitability, availability of transportation and likelihood of relocation.

The overall aim is to obtain a complete inventory of the person's strengths and weaknesses. The result should be a problem list that is then related to what services are needed to restore and maintain the greatest possible independence and the choices-of-living arrangements as preferred by the older person.

THE MULTIDISCIPLINARY TEAM

For a multidisciplinary team to be effective, all members must accept that none has all the answers and all are dependent to various extents on the knowledge of the others. The whole is greater than the sum of its parts. Most teams, therefore, will need to give thought as to their method of working to produce optimal results with the smallest expenditure of time.

This is important, since the aggregate team is an expensive commodity. There are many problems associated with disciplines working together. A clear statement of individual responsibilities and the method for reporting back must be made. In general, the team must define the problems for each old person and arrange appropriate plans of action, which, in turn, must be followed up. The constant objective must be to maximize choice for the individual person rather than to make decisions for them. At the same time realities must be maintained and the position of carers also considered. Communication of the recommendations to the patient and carer is very important as well as to the primary-care physician and team if they are not part of the actual assessment.

The composition of the assessment team will vary according to circumstances. The core members are likely to be a physician, a nurse and a social worker. Additional members may include a physiotherapist, an occupational therapist and a speech therapist. Others who may participate from time to time include a psychogeriatrician and a psychologist. Occasionally, opinions will be sought by and from other specialists. Final recommendations are usually made at case conferences and when these have taken place, it is very important that communication of the findings be made to all the people involved in the care of the old person.

THE PLACE OF ASSESSMENTS IN OVERALL HEALTH AND SOCIAL CARE

The Kellogg Working Party (1987) pointed out that the whole concept of multidisciplinary geriatric assessment will be successfully implemented only if it is integrated into, or has close liaison with, the rest of the health system. This necessity calls for more education and understanding about the nature of geriatric care and the contribution of each professional discipline to the overall care of an elderly person. It will probably need a revision of the current financial barriers to assessment at each point where it is necessary. The implications of this will vary from country to country, but the evidence is strong that assessments are cost-effective as well as being personally rewarding for the patients and families involved. In view of this, suitable educational and, if needed, legislative steps should be taken to help the integration of multidisciplinary geriatric assessment into the health system.

Although greater understanding exists about assessments, there is need for further research. More needs to be known about subgroups of patients most likely to benefit; what the best package of assessment elements is; how the instruments available can be made more useful; and what is the place of self-assessment. Finally there need to be clear indicators of the effectiveness of assessment programmes so that they can be more scientifically monitored and evaluated.

THE INSTRUMENTS AVAILABLE

Although the Working Party listed five main elements involved in assessment (p. 153), the choice of protocols or schedules for undertaking these is wide and no agreement exists as to the most suitable. The situation is complicated further by the differing needs of research and regular practice, each requiring different instruments. The type of situation in which assessment is needed will also alter the protocol. In primary care, most teams will work out protocols that will satisfy their particular needs. Some ideas have already been considered when describing anticipatory care. Normally a protocol should encompass physical, mental, social and environmental status. Functional activity is also important when undertaking assessments. In the author's initial screening assessments, effective health was used as such an assessment. Mental assessments can be done at a simple level, but a well-validated and not-difficult-to-undertake assessment is that designed by Pattie and Gilleard (1979) and published as the Clifton Assessment Procedures for the Elderly (CAPE). It has the advantage of a scale so that monitoring of mental function can taken place. It is divided into a cognitive-assessment scale and a behaviour-rating scale that allow dependency grades to be made and these can be linked to appropriate care.

Williams' rings (Williams, 1986)

In undertaking a social assessment of an old person, it is easy to limit it to a consideration of social history and social status. This would include support networks, financial status, services used, etc. It is very important, however, also to include a functional assessment of social performance. This means consideration of activities of daily living and out of this, three levels of activity have emerged:

1. sociability, which describes activities outside the home
2. domestic, which describes activities inside the home
3. personal, which describes tasks specific to the individual

These have usually been considered separately and the dynamic relationship between the three levels of activity have not been appreciated. If they are seen as three concentric rings surrounding the person, the outer ring represents sociability, the social interaction with the outside world, the middle ring represents the basic activities to preserve domestic equilibrium and the inner ring represents necessities for personal autonomy (see Fig. 14.1).

Out of this concept emerges a model that can be very useful in undertaking assessment of functional status. The outer ring of sociability contains the largest number of possibilities. Elderly people differ in the extent

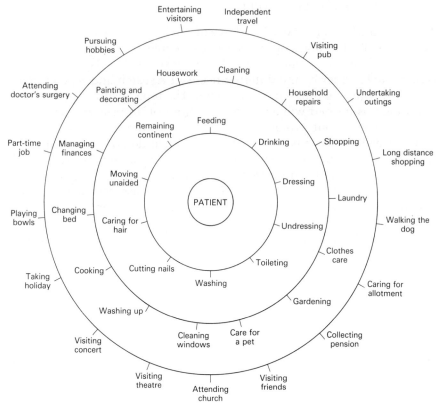

Figure 14.1 Social-performance levels (elderly persons)

of their social involvement outside the home and this is illustrated by the wide variety of the activities shown. It is not expected that each old person will undertake every activity, but they are given as examples. The activities fall, however, into the same general domain, and changes in them are significant. Similarly, in the middle and inner rings it is not necessary for the person to perform every task for him/herself (others can sometimes carry out the task), but to function adequately, each ring needs to be intact.

Ageing is not only a physical process, but also a social one; the natural ageing progression is one of social deterioration. In the model, the process of deterioration generally takes place from the outside inwards. Thus the first sign of breakdown tends to occur at the outer ring. For example, the old person ceases going to the theatre, or to church or stops taking holidays. Signs of a more serious decline occur at the level of the middle ring and herald domestic deterioration. For example, the house is left uncleaned, repairs are not undertaken, cooking becomes hazardous. The final level of social breakdown is at the inner ring where personal tasks are neglected. For example, the person becomes incapable of undertaking bathing, toenail cutting, or attending to make-up or shaving. Sometimes there are early indicators at each level that signal change and are worth identifying. At level one, giving up a hobby or a social activity is an early sign; at level two, shopping is given up, especially if a bus journey is necessary; and at level three, an activity that is commonly the first to cause a problem is bathing unaided.

Other related factors are important when considering the dynamics of social decline between the three levels. There is a gradual deterioration in social ability associated with the ageing process and this commonly takes place over a long period, often with intervening stable intervals. Illness, either physical or mental, usually causes an accelerated decline and change in social function tends to take place within a relatively short time. Exceptions would include slowly developing chronic diseases, although even here the decline would be consistent. Again, withdrawal from social activity may reflect temporary and transient difficulties, a period of depression following a bereavement, for instance, rather than the beginning of permanent decline. It is therefore necessary to consider whether the decline in social ability is due to natural ageing or to illness and to ask about the timing of the loss of social function. If the breakdown is recent, it should be regarded in the first place as a social symptom of a medical disorder and this should prompt an investigation of possible mental or physical cause.

To take account of these points, three further factors therefore need introducing into the ring: time, natural ageing and illness. As they involve all three rings it is possible to represent these radially, thus highlighting the fact that the rate of decline differs depending on whether the cause is natural ageing or illness, and emphasizing the need to be alert to the possibilities of treatment. For example, a patient may find it impossible to continue to tend an allotment and this will soon be followed by the inability to take a bus or do local shopping, and eventually bathing and toenail cutting become difficult. All four disabilities may appear within a short time because the same type of back movements are necessary for each of the tasks. Thus improvement of back mobility could restore functional ability at all three levels.

A complementary model (see Fig. 14.2) demonstrates the type of input usually necessary to restore equilibrium when deterioration in social function has occurred at each level. As deterioration progresses towards the centre new services are needed to augment those already necessary because of breakdown at the outer levels. Thus it is possible to restore a ring by providing appropriate additional assistance; for example, difficulty with bathing may lead to deterioration at the level of the inner

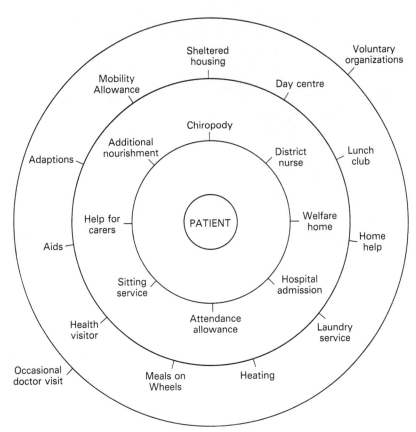

Figure 14.2 Social-input levels (elderly persons)

ring, but bath aids supplied in time could restore independence. Again radial factors come into play. The reason for the loss of the social function should be explored, especially if it has occurred within a short time. Attention to physical and mental causes may mean that additional support is unnecessary. What is important at all levels is the informal networks that support old people and are quite distinct from statutory and voluntary help. The informal network is wider than simply the caring relatives, and is important for maintaining old people in the community and arresting their decline.

Uses of the model

In acute situations where several problems co-exist, the model is helpful in determining the level of social functioning of an elderly patient and the relevance to illness of any decline in function. Decisions may be influenced by understanding the time scale of the deterioration. In continuing care, a record of social ability and the rate of decline are important in monitoring the overall condition. In anticipatory care, it is possible to review the social decline so these steps can be taken at an early stage to introduce appropriate help; in this situation the model is a useful screening tool. Finally, the relatives and carers are affected by the patient's social decline and the care provided by them for old people is often brittle. Often social deterioration at level three is enough to finally break the carer's ability to continue and sometimes hospital admission is necessary. Thus a further value of these rings is to anticipate possible carer breakdown; by identifying problems at level three, which indicate carer stress, appropriate help can be introduced.

Value of the model
To summarize, the model has several uses: it provides three social check lists in caring for elderly people; it takes account of the timing of social deterioration; it highlights the place of physical and mental illness in causing or accelerating social decline; it places emphasis on early restoration of function, either by treatment or care input; it can help carers to understand the significance of social deterioration; it is useful for identifying and managing problems earlier; and it takes into account carer tolerance. Because of its emphasis on functional ability, it facilitates independence amongst old people and therefore contributes to the quality of life.

Computerization

It is possible that certain screening instruments are capable of predicting future functional decline. This could make it easier to plan future needs. Little work has been done along these lines and it is likely that microcomputers will be necessary to facilitate these developments. Over the past few years these have been increasingly used in general practice and they have been shown to contribute significantly to the success of screening programmes in areas such as immunization uptake and cervical cytology. By ranking activities used in the Williams' rings model, it is possible to attach numeric values to functional performance. Experiments are currently being undertaken to test the feasibility of this idea, but at present there is no validated method of making predictions as to future patient needs. This may, however, be possible in the future.

REFERENCES

Danish Medical Bulletin Special Supplement Series on Gerontology No 7 (1987) Multidisciplinary Health Assessment of the Elderly. Copies available from

Kellogg International Health and Ageing Program, 1065 Freize Building, University of Michigan, Ann Arbor, Michigan, USA 48109.

Pattie, A.H. and Gilleard, C.J. (1979) *Manual of the Clifton Assessment Procedures for the Elderly (CAPE)*, Hodder and Stoughton, Sevenoaks, Kent.

Williams, E.I (1986) A model to describe social performance levels in elderly people. *J. R. Coll. Gen. Pract.* **36**, 422–3.

15 *Hospital–community interface*

The main division in the provision of health care for elderly people is between primary and secondary care. The movement of a patient across this interface in both directions is facilitated by the family doctor and other members of the primary-care team. When movement is from community to hospital, there are several pathways by which this can take place. When admission is not required, this is normally to an out-patient department, usually by appointment. If the patient is unable to travel to the hospital out-patient department because of illness or immobility, it is possible to ask a consultant to visit the patient at home and this is known as a domiciliary consultation.

When admission is required, this is normally arranged by the patient's general practitioner, although as will be discussed later, there are other possible methods. On discharge, the patient can be followed up at an out-patients department or at a day hospital, which means shared care with the general practitioner. When discharge from hospital and out-patients occurs, the general practitioner and the team are once more completely responsible for the patient's care.

Within this framework there do, however, develop problems. It sometimes takes many weeks to arrange for an out-patient appointment especially in such specialties as orthopaedics where demand is high. Because of problems in the community – and these can include non-availability of general practitioners – the normal admission processes are sometimes bypassed and patients are admitted by self-referral. However, the single most important difficulty has been the discharge of patients back into the community after hospital admission. Because of the importance of an old patient's discharge from hospital and reception into the community, this section is devoted mainly to this particular event. It will be concerned with describing a recent piece of research that has highlighted many of the difficulties and from which new guidelines have emerged to help with the successful resettlement of patients back into the community.

During the past twenty years there has been a regular flow of studies concerned with the process of discharging elderly patients from hospital and most have described difficulties in resettling such patients. One of the features mentioned has been readmission, especially in emergency. Levels have varied, but it has been as high as 18% in the first year.

Attempts have been made to identify factors that might lead to urgent readmission. Graham and Livesley (1983), studying patients readmitted to a department of geriatric medicine, were able to define causes for readmission. These included unavoidable deterioration of the medical condition, inadequate medical treatment, non-compliance and poor re-habilitation. Victor and Vetter (1985), studying readmission amongst a 4% sample of patients discharged from all specialties found that 17% were readmitted within three months. They found no social or demo-graphic characteristics that were associated with early readmission but commented that it was due mainly to relapse of the original illness.

EARLY UNPLANNED READMISSION

There is also evidence that a high proportion of urgent readmissions take place within 28 days. Because of the importance of this phenomenon, a detailed review is necessary. In a study carried out by Williams and Fitton (1988a,b), an examination was made of the process of discharge and emergency readmission within 28 days. It examined readmissions of old people discharged from hospital across the spectrum of specialties. From the study, valuable insights have been gained about the process of both admission and discharge from hospital.

The study was undertaken in a hospital complex in 1985 and involved collecting details of all patients who were admitted and discharged from the hospital who were over 65 years of age during the course of the year. A random sample of patients who had been admitted in an emergency within 28 days of discharge was constructed (the 'study' group) together with a matched sample of patients who were not readmitted (the 'control' group). There were 133 patients in the study group and the same number in the control group. The main source of data collection was from the patients and their principal informal carers. Interviews with hospital sisters also provided supporting data. With the patients' permission, their general practitioners were contacted by letter and a brief questionnaire was enclosed for completion. There were, therefore, four sources of information and the response rates were good.

By far the greatest proportion of patients were discharged on the first occasion to their place of residence. This applied to 76% of those admitted during the project. Sixteen per cent died during the admission and 6% had not been discharged at the end of data collection. Of those discharg-ed, 6% were readmitted within 28 days as an emergency and 3% were admitted within 28 days as a planned readmission. Of the 266 patients who took part in the project, 64% were women and 36% were men. The most common age range for both sexes was between 70 and 80 years, the mean age of the group being 79.0. Because of matching for age, sex and marital status it was not possible to compare the study and control group for these variables. However, the sample was found to have the same distribution as for all patients aged over 65 admitted during the period of the study, so that it is unlikely that these variables had any effect on readmission. They do, however, provide a representative sample of the hospital population.

Social Classes I and II were underrepresented in the sample and Social Classes IV and V were overrepresented. Eighty per cent of the group lived in private accommodation and there was no correlation between type of living accommodation and emergency readmission. Over half lived with other people; of these, two-thirds lived with their spouse. Again there was no difference between study and control patients but this is likely to have been influenced by matching for marital state and the relatively large age distribution within the group. The majority of the group were widowed, and one-third were married. Income in the form of available cash coming into the household each week was a significant factor in relation to emergency readmission. A greater proportion of the study patients' income was below £58 per week.

The way in which patients were admitted initially to hospital was recorded for both groups and for the study group at the second admission (see Table 15.1). There were 11 methods by which patients were admitted to hospital: their own general practitioner or one from the practice, a deputizing-service general practitioner, a district nurse direct, a social worker direct, following a domiciliary visit by a consultant, direct from an out-patient visit, direct from the day hospital, by the family or a friend direct, by the patient direct, transfer from another hospital and pre-arranged carer relief.

At their first admission, significantly more patients in the study group were admitted by the general practitioner than in the control group. They were also more likely to be admitted direct to hospital by their families or self-referral than those in the control group. Control patients were far more likely to be admitted from out-patient departments or day hospitals. It is possible these findings indicate more serious illness in the study group and as the difference is significant, they are pointers to the likelihood of readmission.

Proportions of modes of admission varied little between the first and second admission of the study patients. It is interesting to note that only 36% of the entire group were admitted by their own general practitioner. Almost the same proportion of study patients were admitted by their general practitioners on the first and second occasion. A surprisingly high proportion of patients were admitted by direct arrangements between the hospital and family, friends or self-referral. The proportions in this respect from the study group's first and second admissions were again very similar. Of those admitted by the general practitioner in the study group the first time, 70% were admitted by the general practitioner on the

Table 15.1 Mode of admission of patients at first and second admission

	Own GP	Deputizing service	Via district nurse/social worker direct	Mode of admission Consultant domiciliary visit	Out-patient/ day hospital	Family/ patient direct	Hospital transfer/carer relief	Total
First admission								
Study Number	57	8	10	9	14	28	6	132
%	43	6	8	7	10	20	5	100
Control Number	38	8	14	10	36	19	8	133
%	29	6	10	8	27	14	6	100
Second admission								
Study Number	60	14	13	7	8	30	–	132
%	45	10	10	5	6	23	–	100

Source: Williams and Fitton (1988a)

second admission and of those who were self- or family-admitted in the first admission, 44% did so again on the second admission.

REASONS FOR READMISSION

All the 133 study patients were readmitted in an emergency. A review of each showed that more often, several factors contributed to the re-admission. In each instance it was, however, possible to identify one principal reason, although this was sometimes difficult because two factors seemed to be of nearly equal importance.

There were seven principal reasons for readmission (see Table 15.2). The most common was relapse of the initial medical condition. The criterion used was that the relapse produced a medical situation that necessitated readmission in its own right. The 'new problem' group consisted of 20 patients who developed a new condition that did not relate to the original.

Very many of the readmitted patients had carer problems but in 19 cases it was thought that the reason for readmission was principally carer failure. In only 5 of these cases was the carer a spouse. In the remainder they were other relatives, except for two cases in which the carers were a lodger and a neighbour. Both were described as giving formal care, but they were clearly not reliable in the context of being able to provide consistent and adequate support. Of the 7 people who were readmitted because of complication of the original illness, 5 were orthopaedic and 2

Table 15.2 Principal reasons for unplanned readmission

Reasons for readmission	n	%	Mean age (yrs)	Sex m (n)	f	Lives alone (n)	(%)	Interval between discharge and readmission (days) Median	Range
Relapse of initial illness	67	51	79.9	26	41	30	45	11	1–27
New problem developed	20	15	74.3	5	15	6	30	9	1–20
Carer problems	19	14	79.5	4	15	9	47	7	1–27
Complications of initial illness	7	5	71.0	1	6	4	57	3	1–25
Terminal care	8	6	74.6	5	3	1	12	15	7–27
Medication problems	8	6	79.0	4	4	4	50	8	1–23
Problems with services	4	3	80.0	3	1	3	75	14	4–24
Whole group	133	100	76.9					9	1–27

Source: Williams and Fitton (1988b)

were surgical cases. Most were complications of surgery. Eight patients were readmitted for terminal care; all suffered from neoplastic disease. As would be expected, those who cared for them at home were under severe pressure. In 6 of these cases the carer was a husband or wife who was also elderly and in poor health. The next group was associated with medication failure. It had been expected that problems with medication might feature as a contributory factor rather than as a principal reason for readmission. However, in 8 cases, medication problems directly caused the subsequent readmission. Finally, 4 cases were readmitted directly as a result of failure in formal services. All of them were due to district-nurse failure because of communication breakdown between hospital and community services.

Table 15.2 shows the principal reason for readmission in relation to age, sex and whether the patient lived alone and the mean number of days between discharge and readmission. The median interim between discharge and readmission for the total group of 133 patients was 9 days. This varied according to the reason for readmission. Complications, medication problems and carer problems resulted in quick readmission, whereas unplanned terminal care and problems with services took longer to emerge. Although the numbers were too few to make a definitive statement in this respect they may indicate a trend. The relationship between the patient's sex and the reason for readmission does not appear to be significant. There were high proportions of those living with others among patients who were readmitted with relapse, or a new problem or terminal care. Considering the varying specialties, there was no overall statistically significant difference between the readmission rates for each of these. There were relatively more geriatric medicine patients in the study group but most of the specialties had nearly equal numbers of study and control patients. Orthopaedic surgery was, however, the exception where there were 59% in the control group compared with 41% in the study group.

In nearly every case there were contributory factors that made readmission more likely. The seven principal reasons for readmission have been identified but each of these could also have been a contributory factor. For example, the prime cause could have been a medication problem but relapse and carer difficulties may well have been strong contributory factors. Fifteen contributory factors were identified and are shown in Table 15.3. Carer difficulties stand out clearly as being the most significant in relation to readmission. The practical and emotional strain of caring for an elderly patient who has just been discharged from hospital was very apparent during interviews. Premature discharge, as assessed by study patients and carers, was the second most common contributory factor. In 24 cases the general practitioner was in agreement that the discharge was premature. Other causes for concern were the

Table 15.3 Contributory factors in early unplanned readmission
n = 133 except where stated

Contributory factors	Number	%
Carer problems (*n* = 100)	83	83
Discharge too soon – carer's/patient's opinion	77	58
GP's opinion (n = 83)	26	31
Lack of information from hospital to GP (n = 104)	49	47
Living alone	57	43
Poor health on discharge – carer's/patient's opinion	49	37
Inadequate preparation for discharge	49	37
Incontinence (urinary and faecal)	44	33
Medication problems	39	29
Problems with services	24	18
Relapse of initial illness	18	14
General practitioner's failure to visit	15	11
Very confused: hospital/patient/carer opinion	13	10
New problems developed	4	3
Discharged self	2	2
Complication of initial illness	1	1

Source: Williams and Fitton (1988b)

high level of medication problems, service failure, poor preparation for discharge in terms of assessment, advice and too short notice, failure of notification to general practitioners and/or their subsequent failure to visit patients when discharged. Confusion and incontinence, especially if it were both faecal and urinary, were also factors. Readmitted patients often had more than one contributory factor and sometimes had many. One patient had nine! Problems were not, however, absent in the control group and only a very good carer presence prevented readmission. Some people were readmitted in the fifth and sixth weeks following discharge for much the same reasons as those in the study group and they could easily be classed as emergency early readmission. Problems were more common, however, in the study group and often significantly so, as is shown in Table 15.4.

Apart from direct and contributory reasons for readmission there were some other statistically significant differences between the study and the control group. These included:

Low income
High level of previous admission
Where a district nurse or social worker was already visiting
Admission by their own general practitioner
Carers who had concern about their own health
Carers who had a high frustration level

Table 15.4 Comparison between study and control patients regarding factors that would contribute to readmission

Problem	Study no	Study %	Control no	Control %	Significance		
1. Carer's problems: (n = 193: Study = 100 Control = 93)							
health affected	54	54	34	37	$X^2 = 5$	1df	p<0.05
frustration and restriction	67	67	34	37	$X^2 = 16.7$	1df	p<0.0005
difficulty with communication	31	31	13	14	$X^2 = 7$	1df	p<0.01
2. Too early discharge GP opinion (n = 179: Study = 83 Control = 96)	26	31	11	12	$X^2 = 14.4$	1df	p<0.001
3. Poor health on discharge Ward sister opinion (n = 265: Study = 132 Control = 133)	13	10	5	4	$X^2 = 9.25$	2df	p<0.01
4. No advice given at discharge (n = 263: Study = 130 Control = 133)	66	51	43	32	$X^2 = 9.2$	1df	p=0.002
5. Incontinence (urinary or faecal) (n = 265: Study = 132 Control = 133)	22	17	16	12	$X^2 = 1.2$	1df	NS
6. Problems with medication after discharge (n = 266: Study = 133 Control = 133)	42	31	50	38	$X^2 = 1.1$	1df	NS
7. Problems with services after discharge (n = 266: Study = 133 Control = 133)	52	39	44	33	$X^2 = 1.0$	1df	NS
8. No GP visit after discharge (n = 260: Study = 128 Control = 132)	36	28	50	38	$X^2 = 3$	1df	NS
9. No discharge notice to GP (n = 207: Study = 101 Control = 106)	30	30	8	8	$X^2 = 15.4$	1df	p=0.0001

Source: Williams and Fitton (1988b)

Carers engaged in personal tasks for the patient, for example, washing
  and dressing
Faecal incontinence
Communication problems between patient and carer
Poor mobility

The following list shows factors for which statistical significance was
nearly reached:

Admission to a department of geriatric medicine
Over five items of medication prescribed on discharge
Discharge late in the day
No transport of the patient's own
Carers with long-standing illnesses
Carers who had to do the housework for the patient
Carers who were not spouses
Carers with family problems of their own
Carers who had experienced life problems in the previous year
Living in the present house for a relatively short time
Poor general health

An assessment was made as to whether readmission was preventable.
It was noted that readmission was likely to have been avoided if more
effective action had been taken in one or more of five areas. These were:
preparation for and timing of the discharge, attention to the needs of the
carer, timing and adequate information to the GP and subsequent action
by the GP, sufficient and prompt nursing and social-service support and,
finally, management of medication. It was considered that in about 60%
of the cases, readmission would have been avoided if proper arrangements had been made in these areas.

The overall impression was that patients were receiving adequate
services before the first admission. The high level of these indicated the
vulnerability of the patients. In general, the study group had more help
than the control group probably because of the severity of illness. The
range of the services is shown in Table 15.5. A substantial number of
patients had services organized for them on leaving hospital. These were
not necessarily the same services that had been present before admission.
Sometimes patients refused services at this time mainly for financial
reasons. Just over half of the study group had a district nurse arranged at
discharge; half of these were new services and the remainder were
reinstated. Just over one-third of control patients had a district nurse
arranged, two-thirds of which were new services. The result was a net
increase in district nursing for the whole group. The level of district-
nursing service increased significantly with age.

About half of the study group and slightly under half of the control

Table 15.5 Provision of services on first admission and after first discharge

Service	Group	% of patients receiving service on first admission	% of patients receiving service on first discharge	increase/ decrease (%)
District nurse	Study	40	51	+ 11
	Control	25	39	+ 14
Social worker	Study	23	35	+ 12
	Control	10	16	+ 6
Meals on wheels	Study	10	20	+ 10
	Control	9	16	+ 7
Day centre	Study	11	18	+ 7
	Control	8	17	+ 9
Home help	Study	35	40	+ 5
	Control	30	35	+ 5
Physiotherapy	Study	4	3	− 1
	Control	3	6	+ 3
Health visitor	Study	18	14	− 4
	Control	14	14	=
Chiropodist	Study	35	6	− 29
	Control	41	18	− 25

Source: Williams and Fitton (1988a)

group had home-help service, most of which was reinstated. The use of home-help services also increased significantly with age and also with living alone and absence of a carer. A social worker was arranged for about one-third of the study patients but for very few of the control group. Other services were organized for relatively few patients. In all circumstances, those who were very old, lived alone, were in poor general health, were confused, had poor mobility or were incontinent were the most likely to have services arranged.

Problems were, however, present with the services. Excluding general-practitioner services, 36% of the total group complained of difficulties with formal carers. The variety of problems experienced was great and many patients seemed to have had more than one type of problem. These are shown in Table 15.6. There were more problems in the study group but nevertheless, the level was not significantly different between that and the control group. The problems were basically of three types: no arrangements; delay in starting the service; inadequate service to meet the needs. These occurred throughout the different services but the most important failure was when nursing services were deficient. The most serious situation was when nobody turned up to the patient's home after discharge, and this was always due to communication failure. Also, administrative problems sometimes caused deficiencies. In 18% of the

Table 15.6 Problems with services

	Study		Control	
	No	*%*	*No*	*%*
Inadequate provision of services (district nurse, social worker combined)	18	34	17	39
Delay in start after discharge: (a) District nurse	10	19	5	11
(b) Other (social worker, home help, meals on wheels, occupational therapist)	9	17	15	34
Inadequate hospital preparation and lack of arrangements	10	19	1	2
Personality clashes	3	6	1	2
Housing/finance	2	4	5	11
Total	52		44	

Source: Williams and Fitton (1988a)

readmitted group, service failure was considered to be a strong contributory factor to readmission.

These experiences show that despite reasonable levels of service provision, problems can still occur. Communication problems certainly need attention. It would seem that someone in the community should assess the needs of the patient as soon as discharge occurs. Delay in instituting services is very important to the lives of the patients, particularly when they live alone, and, of course, to the carers.

Notice of discharge either by a discharge note or formal letter was never received by the general practitioner for 18% of the total group. There was also delay in receiving notification even when this was eventually received. The doctors heard about the discharge within the first week in only 66% of cases. There was dissatisfaction among general practitioners about both the information received from the hospital and the delay in receiving such notice. Considering general-practitioner visits after discharge of the whole group, 67% received a visit from a general practitioner at some stage, but post-discharge visits were most likely to have been initiated by the patients and their families. GPs were most likely to visit patients who had informal carers or who were very old.

Patients were asked whether they were satisfied with their general practitioner. Nearly three-quarters were, but some were very dissatisfied. The carers, when asked the same question, were more critical. Both volunteered information about the doctor's handling of the discharge procedure. The main criticisms were when no follow-up visiting was arranged, especially to housebound patients. They also commented about some general practitioners' unsympathetic manner and sometimes poor management. Clearly, a code of practice is needed about informing the GP about discharge of an elderly patient and the way in which GPs should respond to the discharge. Although it is realized that some discharged patients will not need a home visit, it is probable that some contact is still necessary at the doctor's surgery to review needs and to discuss problems. Attitudes towards patients who are old are clearly important in determining outcome and patient satisfaction.

During the study some very interesting information was gathered about the carers of patients discharged from hospital. It is possible that what was found was an indication of the difficulties experienced by carers of old people in general. Of the total group of patients, 18% had no identifiable formal carer and this in itself poses immediate problems in the community. The majority of carers were over 60 years old themselves, and some of them were very old indeed. One-third were men and two-thirds were women. A quarter of the carers did not live with the patient for whom they were caring. The stress of caring for an older patient was very apparent. Nearly half of the total group said their health had been affected by the tasks. There was also a considerable amount of frustration. Many carers felt restricted and tied because of patients' continuing needs. Some carers said that their own family life had been destroyed at the expense of meeting the patients' needs and this happened especially when the carers did not live with the patients. The carers often felt depressed and fatigued and had experienced problems 'with their nerves'. They commented on the unremitting pressure on them and time-consuming nature of the job of attending to the patients' needs.

Carers also mentioned problems associated with dissatisfaction with the hospital's management of the patient's medical condition and follow-up support. They were frustrated by the differences between their perception of the severity of the patient's condition and the hospital staff's assessment. They felt the hospital were underassessing the severity of the patient's condition and the result was that they felt they were deprived of much needed care and support. Carers were very often coping with personal tasks for patients such as dressing, bathing and washing and also, in many cases, were having to deal with household tasks. Some of this care had been going on for many years. The whole problem was often aggravated by patients' incontinence, which was found to be a hard problem to tolerate. In a few cases the carers were concerned about the fact that the patients were neglecting themselves or were at risk of accidents or misuse of prescribed drugs. A few carers had to contend with irresponsible behaviour.

Carers are a very important group with real needs in the community. They need information about the patient from both the hospital and the community workers. This must include details of the medical condition and treatment, what is a likely outcome and what is the general assessment of the patient's condition and abilities. Also, there must be an assessment of the carers' needs themselves. Perhaps additional home help is required. It is tempting to think that when there is a carer present, no additional help is needed. Sometimes, especially in the first few weeks after discharge, financial help may also be needed and an attendance allowance should be applied for.

Nearly 85% of the total group went home on some medication and nearly 30% went home with more than four items. The older the patient, the more likely it was that medication was given on discharge, although they were less likely to be given more than four items. Medication was used as directed in only 45% of cases. The largest proportion of prescriptions were drugs for the cardiovascular, respiratory and central nervous systems. About one-third of the group had problems with medication. There were many types. Medication was sometimes inappropriate, as, for example, the patient who was kept on thyroxine despite coronary artery disease and severe asthma. Patient confusion was also a problem. Several examples were seen of patients who were too confused to understand their medication. Patients occasionally were actually taking the tablets in the wrong doses despite verbal and written instructions to the contrary. There were frequent examples of cases where neither patient nor carer understood what the tablets were actually being taken for. Carers confessed to having tried tablets themselves to see if they could determine the effect. Sometimes instructions on the container did not agree with the verbal instructions given at the hospital. Necessary drugs were not given to the patients at discharge or the wait for them to be dispensed was too long, so the patient left without any supplies. There were also problems with patients' eyesight that made it difficult for them to see the labels and also to tell which were the different types of tablets. Patients were sometimes not confident that changes made by the hospital in relation to treatment that they had been previously taking were in fact correct and so reverted to the previous dosage. Sometimes medication was too difficult to handle; for example, one patient found a salbutamol inhaler impossible to use. Some of these problems were serious and involved early readmission.

MEDICATION GUIDELINES

The study highlights the fact that discharge from hospital can be associated with medication problems. There should be clear guidelines available to minimize these difficulties. These could include:

1. Counsel patients and carers before discharge about medication;
2. Give appropriately labelled and easy-to-handle bottles and containers;

3. Give a ten-day supply of a drug with instructions to let the GP know of the need for a repeat prescription at an early point;
4. Give verbal and written instructions to carers, especially when patients are confused;
5. Take account of the patient's health before dispensing so that problems associated with confusion, arthritis, immobility can be foreseen;
6. Have a check list to go through with the patient about important instructions;
7. Give early notification to the general practitioner.

GENERAL GUIDELINES FOR DISCHARGE

It is clear that at such an important point in a patient's life as a discharge from hospital, clear guidelines should be available as to how this should be managed, both for the community and the hospital. The following are suggested for the hospital:

Assess home circumstances;
Check that carers exist at home;
Ascertain that discharge is appropriate;
Assess the patient's ability to self-care at home;
Give adequate warning to relatives and carers;
Arrange transport so that the patient can get home during the day time;
Go through a drug check list;
Make sure that appropriate advice is understood;
Confirm arrangements for services;
Check that some professional in the community knows that the patient is being discharged;
Ring the GP surgery with brief details;
Beware of special circumstances where early readmission is more likely; these would include:
low-income groups
where the patient has been in hospital often before
where the illness has been severe
where the patient's general condition is poor, especially where confusion, immobility and incontinence occur
where patients were admitted by the general practitioner
where the carer is in poor health or has other commitments.

Similar guidelines should be followed by those responsible in the community. Each patient who is discharged should be visited by someone from the practice within 48 hours to check carer presence and needs, medication, services, general condition and follow-up requirements. Also, it is necessary to check on general advice and support, especially in circumstances where readmission may be more likely.

REFERENCES

Graham, H. and Livesley, B. (1983) Can readmissions to a geriatric medical unit be prevented? *Lancet*, **i**, 404–6.
Victor, C. and Vetter, N.J. (1985) The early readmission of the elderly to hospital. *Age and Ageing*, **52**, (i), 79–84.
Williams, E.I. and Fitton, F. (1988a) Factors affecting early unplanned readmission of elderly hospital patients. Report to the North West Regional Health Authority Research Committee. Unpublished.
Williams, E.I. and Fitton, F. (1988b) Factors affecting early unplanned readmission of elderly hospital patients. *Br. Med. J.*, **297**, 784–7.

16 *The old person in family medicine*

Clinical aspects

The medical community care of old people in the United Kingdom largely takes place in health centres or in doctors' surgeries. In other countries there are variations, but the essential processes of care remain the same. For non-ambulant patients, care is available in their own homes, in nursing or rest homes and in welfare homes. The number of old people using these services make them an important part of primary care. This chapter will consider the pattern of care provided and some clinical aspects.

Old persons attend a doctor with a wide variety of different problems and receive a wide variety of treatments, investigations and referrals. A good deal is known about people referred to the hospital service, but relatively little about the vast majority who receive medical treatment in the community. Drawing on data collected during a study in primary care Wilkin and Williams (1986) began to fill this gap. The research was based on information collected from two hundred GPs in all consultations occurring on a representative sample of fifteen working days. Data on some 90 thousand consultations were analysed, of which 20 thousand were with people over 65 years of age (Wilkin *et al.*, 1984).

DISTRIBUTION OF CONSULTATIONS BY AGE

The distribution of consultations by age was compared with the distribution of the total population of the study area, as indicated in the 1981 census; a predictable pattern was observed. The age group 0–14 made up 20% of the total population, but only 17% of consultations. At the other end of the age spectrum, this was reversed, so that those aged 75 years or over made up 6% of the population, but 8% of consultations. However, there was a gradual increase from middle age to old age in terms of numbers consulting general practitioners. There was no evidence of a sharp change at the age of 65. The overall pattern was similar to that reported in the National Morbidity Study for 1971/2 which showed a total of 17% of consultations with patients in the over-65 age group, compared with 19% in the study (Wilkin and Williams, 1986). This may indicate that the contribution of elderly people to the work of the general practitioner is increasing as the number of elderly people in the population rises.

DISEASE CATEGORIES

Data was available from the study of the relative importance of different diagnostic categories and these changed sharply with age in the adult population (see Table 16.1). Circulatory and musculoskeletal disorders became progressively more important with increasing age, whilst infectious disease, mental disease, genitourinary disease, skin disorders and accidents all decreased in proportion to the total case mix. Such change was even more pronounced than is suggested in the table because the presentation concealed considerable variations within the broad International Classification of Diseases (ICD) categories (WHO, 1978). Thus, not only was there an increase in the proportion of endocrine and metabolic diseases, but within this category the proportion of consultations for diabetes mellitus increased. For the 15–54 age group, 19% of diagnoses in the category 'endocrine and metabolic disorders' were for diabetes, but for the 74-and-over age group this figure had risen to 54%. Although the relative importance of psychiatric disorders declines with age, GPs were dealing with more chronic problems in elderly people. Amongst the 85-

Table 16.1 Diagnostic categories by age group (percentages)

ICD category	Age group				Total
	15–54	*55–64*	*65–74*	*75+*	
Infectious and parasitic	7.7	3.4	2.9	2.3	5.7
Neoplasms	0.9	2.3	2.7	3.1	1.6
Endocrine, nutritional and metabolic	2.3	3.5	3.3	3.1	2.7
Blood	0.7	0.6	1.3	2.1	0.9
Mental	9.3	9.3	7.6	7.3	8.9
Central nervous system	6.1	6.6	6.9	7.1	6.4
Circulatory system	4.6	19.7	24.4	25.9	12.2
Respiratory system	14.5	15.7	15.2	12.0	14.5
Digestive system	4.9	5.7	5.1	5.0	5.1
Genitourinary	6.6	3.1	2.5	2.4	5.0
Skin	6.0	3.8	3.4	3.2	5.0
Musculoskeletal	7.6	13.0	12.6	13.3	9.8
Signs and symptoms	2.3	2.3	2.5	4.0	2.5
Accidents, injury, etc.	6.7	4.2	3.4	3.7	5.5
Supplementary	19.0	6.8	6.1	5.4	13.7
Total number (100%)	45 846	12 454	11 154	8278	77 732

Source: Wilkin and Williams (1986)

plus age group, 52% of psychiatric diagnoses were for dementia and only 22% for anxiety or depression. For respiratory disorders, minor respiratory-tract infection became progressively less important with age, whilst acute and chronic bronchitis became more important. Bronchitis accounted for 14% of diagnoses in this category in the 15–54 age group, and 50% for the 75-and-over age group. In the category of 'signs and symptoms', 36% of the over-75-year olds were described as suffering from senility or senescence. Interestingly, the proportion of consultations for marital and social problems was low for all age groups. There was no evidence that a GP recorded more social problems amongst older patients. The proportion of patients with more than one diagnosis increased from 14% in the 15–54 age group to 20% for those aged 55 to 64, 23% for the 65–74 age group and 24% for those aged over 75. Older patients were therefore more commonly presenting to general practitioners with a complex interaction of health problems.

The types of problems presented to the GP according to age reveal predictable patterns (Wilkin *et al.*, 1987). Coughs, colds and sore throats were 45% of all symptoms presented by young children (0–5 years), but only 14% of those presented by old people. In contrast, muscular aches and pains constituted less than 10% of symptoms amongst children and teenagers (0–17 years) and 23% amongst elderly people. Skin infections and irritation were most common amongst teenagers (15% of all symptoms) and least common in elderly people (5% of all symptoms). Not only do these patterns reflect possible variations in the prevalence of these symptoms at different ages, they also reflect attitudes towards symptoms when they occur. Willingness to tolerate particular symptoms is dependent on a wide range of social factors and on expectations of what is normal, and these turn out to be age related. Thus, for example, parents are understandably concerned about the possible effects of coughs and colds in small children although they may think nothing of the same symptoms themselves. Older people who may be suffering from symptoms of long-term chronic illness would be less likely to go to the GP with apparently minor symptoms.

PATTERNS OF CARE

In the light of these changes in the case mix mentioned previously, it is hardly surprising that differences were found in the pattern of care provided for different age groups (see Table 16.2). The proportion of new consultations (patient-initiated rather than doctor-initiated) declined with age so that amongst the very old, two-thirds of all consultations were for follow-up care. However, this change did not occur sharply at the age of 65. There was a steady upward trend in the proportion of follow-up work done with increasing age. At the same time the proportion of consultations conducted in the patient's home increased, but in this case, there was a

Table 16.2 The pattern of care as a percentage of all consultations in the study population in one year

Age group			Percentage			
	New cases	Home visits	Prescription	Lab-test	Consultant referral	Other referral
15–54	55	5	67	5	7	2
55–64	39	8	74	3	6	1
65–74	37	20	80	3	6	2
75+	33	47	75	2	6	3

Source: Wilkin and Williams (1986)

marked difference between the 55–64 age group and the 65–74 age group, and again for the 75-plus age group. This continued into the very old 85-plus age group, where two-thirds of consultations were home visits. Older patients (55 plus) were more likely to receive a prescription than young adults, but this pattern did not continue into the 75-plus age group. This may reflect an increase in the level of surveillance and follow-up for very elderly people, since such consultations often required no further treatment. However, often the complex multiple pharmacology amongst elderly patients might suggest a need for more investigation. It was therefore surprising to find that laboratory utilization declined from 5% of all consultations in the 15–55 age group to 2% for the over-75 age group. Although elderly people are generally known to be heavy users of hospital services, there is no evidence of greater propensity for GPs to refer older patients. Indeed, referrals to consultants declined very slightly with age in contrast with referrals to district nurses and social services, which increased, but even amongst the 75-plus age group, referrals to all other agencies combined to only half the level of those to consultants.

Variations in patterns of care

There was an enormous variation between GPs. Fig. 16.1 shows consultation rates and indicates the extent of this variation. The overall rate for elderly people was 4.6 consultations per year compared with 2.9 for those aged less than 65 years, but for more than a quarter of GPs the elderly consultation rate was less than 3 contacts per year. A similar proportion saw their elderly patients more than 6 times a year. Home visits were equally varied. Of GPs, 16% did less than 5 home visits per week whilst 15 per cent did more than 30. Referral rates also showed similar variation. The average rate was 6%, but 13% of GPs had rates higher than 10% and a similar proportion had rates below 2%.

Several important findings came out of this study. Whilst it is almost a truism to say that old age does not begin at 65, the very fact that this administrative dividing line is usually adopted for practical and research purposes tends to generate a perception of old age as a discrete pheno-

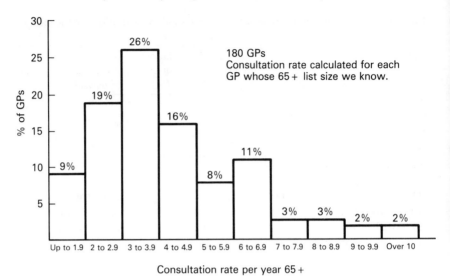

Figure 16.1 Consultation rate for patients 65+ years

menon. Comparisons between elderly people (65-plus) and the rest of the population appear to reveal sharp differences, but the data show a more gradual transition in which 55–64 age groups have more in common with the 65–74 than with the younger adult population.

The general point can be made that ageing is a biological, psychological and social process that is only turned into a discrete entity by administrative regulations, for instance retirement age, additional payments for GPs and specialist hospital services. Whilst there are reasonable grounds for such rules, there is no necessity to reinforce the negative stereotypes of old age that are all too common already. At least in primary care it should be possible to treat ageing as the variable process the evidence clearly shows it to be, and treating patients as individuals in the wider contexts of their total lives.

The pattern of general-practitioner care for elderly patients clearly changes with increasing age. More follow-up work is done with elderly patients; they are visited more often in their homes and more referrals are made to nursing and social services. However, less investigative work is done and there is no change in the number of referrals to consultants. The variations in the pattern of care provided for old people is, however, very striking. Different GPs clearly have different views of what is appropriate for their patients. Old people can experience gross differences in primary health care if they happen to be registered with different doctors. Not only does this have implications for old people themselves, but also for the rest of the services. Individual people do not necessarily have similar access to specialist services through the referral system. Nothing is known about the effectiveness of GP care or whether it is influenced by this variation. A higher referral rate, for instance, may not mean a higher standard of care. The fact remains that 94% of all people over the age of 65 still live in their own homes and receive their medical care from general practitioners.

RECORD KEEPING

Good care of old people requires accurate and appropriate records. It is desirable that on every patient's sixty-fifth birthday a review of the records should take place, discarding redundant documents and starting a new system. An age/sex register of patients over 65 is essential in planning preventive and anticipatory care. Some practices also keep a register of the attendance of an old person with either doctor, nurse or health visitor and for repeat prescriptions, so that information is available about those who do not attend. It is likely that non-attenders will be in good health, but it is a good idea for a health visitor to visit them occasionally. Admissions and discharges of old people to hospital, welfare and nursing home can also be recorded in the register and this enables more effective care to be given during these periods (see Fig. 16.2).

A good idea is also to maintain a disease or disability register. This can be done for the over-65 population or, indeed, for the whole practice. The number of disabilities recorded may vary between ten and fifty, but it is probably wise to limit the number to a relatively small number of important conditions. This is so that the task does not become too daunting! Examples would include diabetes mellitus, dementia, vision problems, immobility due to arthritis, stroke and heart failure. These registers are particularly useful when undertaking an audit of care for particular diseases.

It is interesting to consider what proportion of patients in a practice are disabled. In a questionnaire survey of general practitioners carried out in 1983, the author found that most of the responding doctors thought that it was less than 15% and that most of these disabled were in the over-65 age group. The doctors were asked to state which type of patients they considered to be disabled. Table 16.3 lists these with the percentage of doctors mentioning each category. Included in the group 'Other' was disability caused by social impairment, whether environmental, economic, cultural or educational. The list gives some idea of the type of categories that could be included in a disability register.

The record system used by most GPs is the 'Lloyd George' envelope. This is highly unsatisfactory, but the move to A4 records has been slow and relatively few GPS have this system. The review at 65 years may be an opportunity for changing to A4 records so that elderly people in the practice have this type of record. Clearly, the letters and investigations need to be filed separately in the notes in date order. Problem lists, both active and inactive, are very useful. An up-to-date therapy list is also

DOCTOR: A Brown

DATE OF BIRTH	*PATIENT'S NAME*	JAN			FEB			MAR			APR			MAY			JUNE			JULY			AUG			SEPT			OCT			NOV			DEC		
		S	P	V	S	P	V	S	P	V	S	P	V	S	P	V	S	P	V	S	P	V	S	P	V	S	P	V	S	P	V	S	P	V	S	P	V
1.1.02	John Smith				11		1	11					1			1	1							1			1				1			1			1
1.1.02	Mary Jones	11			11			1					1			1		1				1	1				1				1			1			1

S = Surgery attendance
P = Repeat prescription
V = Home visit

Figure 16.2 Patient Register

Table 16.3 Doctors' perception of disability – conditions mentioned spontaneously in response to the question 'Which specific groups of patients do you regard as disabled?'

Disability	Extent of disability	Doctors (%)
Blindness	Complete or partial	77.3
Mental problem	Congenital or acquired incapacitating mental illness	76.6
Mobility problem	Arthritis of all types	76.6
Deafness	Complete or partial	64.1
Cardiovascular disease	Failure, angina, claudication	56.3
Respiratory disease	Obstructive airways, bronchitis	52.3
Children	With congenital defect	50.8
Stroke		51.6
Neurological disease	Multiple sclerosis, Parkinsonism	42.2
Amputation		33.6
Effects of trauma		21.1
Incontinence	Urinary or faecal	5.5
Other	Included diabetes, epilepsy, stoma, speech defect, social problems	39.8

Source: Williams (1983)

essential, especially when repeat prescriptions are being issued. Many practices have treatment cards that the patient holds. These have many advantages especially where several workers are involved. They do, however, need to be kept up to date and accurate. An important inclusion in the records is detail of any assessments that have been carried out and a provision for updating these assessments. Who should have access to the note system is often debated and patients themselves also have rights in this matter. Most practices would expect key health workers to use and contribute to the records. The introduction of computers into practices has made many of these tasks easier. New developments in methods of payment to GPs, particularly in respect of their elderly patients, may make a computer essential.

PRINCIPLES OF MEDICATION

Most doctors are aware of the risks of prescribing large numbers of drugs for elderly patients and they are also aware of the demand from some old people for these drugs to alleviate multiple symptomatology. The pressure on the doctor to give symptomatic treatment can be quite considerable. At the same time, most doctors, nurses and social workers have had the experience of finding an old person at home with a large number of bottles of tablets on the mantlepiece, only to discover when moving into the kitchen or bathroom an equally large number of bottles on shelves and in cabinets. The old person is all too often unaware of what the tablets are for; many of them have been in the house for a long time and the taking of them is frequently quite irrational and haphazard. This is not confined to patients at home. When visiting welfare homes or private nursing homes, it is remarkable to see the long lists pinned up in the office of drugs that each old person is taking or supposed to be taking. There is thus a situation where large quantities and types of medicines are prescribed for old people, and it is constantly necessary to review the policy of drug therapy for elderly people. Ivan Illich (1975), in his criticism of the medical profession, points out that one out of every five patients admitted to a typical research hospital acquires iatrogenic disease, often as a complication of drug therapy. How much similar disease is being caused in the community by careless prescribing is unknown.

A recently published book by Ann Cartwright and Christopher Smith (1988) describes a study that looked at the medicines prescribed for and taken by a nationally representative sample of elderly people. An increasing proportion of all prescribed medicines now go to people aged over 65 (see Fig. 16.3). In 1985, the most recent year for which figures are available, the proportion of elderly people in the population was 18% and they received 39% of the prescription items dispensed. While the numbers of all prescription items for all ages increased by 8% between 1977 and 1984, there was a slight fall in the prescribing for the non-elderly age group. Larger changes were seen for medicines in certain therapeutic groups (see Table 16.4). It is interesting to note that for all ages the number of prescriptions for sedatives and tranquillizers decreased substantially.

The study found that on average, elderly people were taking just under two prescribed medicines; roughly one-third were taking none, one-third one or two and one-third three or more. Encouragingly nearly three-fifths of the study population regarded their health for their age as excellent or good. These old people understood at least something of the purpose of nearly all the prescribed medicines they were taking and said they found most of them very helpful. The majority, three-quarters, of the elderly people took their prescribed medicines as advised. However, the study did identify some discouraging features, particularly in the information that old people were given about their medicines; also the record keeping of doctors and the supervision that was given to the patients was not satisfactory. Labelling of the prescribed medicines was also found to be unsuitable in form. Cartwright and Smith (1988) gave some specific recommendations that included the need to improve record keeping and the greater involvement of pharmacists in improving effectiveness of prescribing. More education for trainee general practitioners and medical students was advocated. They concluded that labelling of medicines should be improved and that it would be helpful if written information was given to patients about their medicines.

In old age, changes occur in certain physiological functions that can affect the action of drugs in the body. Absorption normally takes place

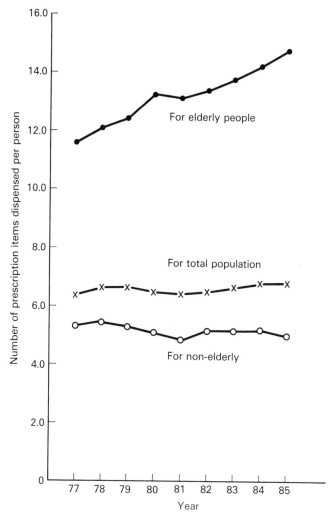

Figure 16.3 Recent trends in prescribing (from Cartwright and Smith, 1988)

from the gastrointestinal tract and ageing may reduce the blood flow to these areas and the number of absorbing cells. There is no direct evidence, however, that absorption is seriously reduced in old age. Metabolism normally occurs in the liver, where drugs are broken down to inactive forms prior to excretion via the kidney. Some drugs are excreted unchanged. In old age, both the liver and kidney can become less efficient in undertaking these processes, and this can lead to slower elimination of drugs from the body and they can therefore remain active for longer periods. This natural physiological ageing process can be augmented by disease. Renal and hepatic illness can reduce drug elimination, as can general conditions such as heart failure or dehydration. Reduction in

Table 16.4 Some trends in prescribing by therapeutic class

Therapeutic class	Number of preparations dispensed			Proportional change (%)
	1977	*1980*	*1984*	*1977–84*
Sedatives and tranquillizers	20 836	18 920	13 622	−35
Hypnotics	14 015	13 626	13 471	−4
Analgesics – minor	17 578	17 409	17 958	+2
Antidepressants	6 715	6 263	6 185	−8
Preparations acting on the heart	12 763	16 922	19 851	+56
Diuretics	15 549	19 538	21 700	+40
Antihypertensives	5 603	6 081	7 972	+42
Preparations prescribed for rheumatism	13 595	15 839	17 915	+32
All other prescriptions	167 701	168 809	180 138	+7
All groups	295 656	303 334	320 543	+8

Source: Cartwright and Smith (1988)

overall body size associated with old age may affect the distribution of drugs in the body. Tissues may alter in their response to certain drugs, a good example being barbiturates, where sedative effect on the brain may be increased. Old people, therefore, can be expected to be more sensitive to the effect of drugs and suffer more often from side-effects. Drug interactions of a synergistic or antagonistic nature may also be increased.

It is hard to determine in an individual patient whether physiological changes will have occurred sufficiently to cause increased liability of side-effects or incorrect dosage. Actual chronological age may outstrip biological age and an old person may retain perfectly efficient physiological mechanisms. Nevertheless, the danger must be appreciated and watch kept for possible overtreatment. Not all drugs are affected by these changes. In general, preparations used as replacement therapy need to be given in normal doses and, indeed, there is sometimes the danger of undertreatment. For instance, in thyroid deficiency, it might be that too low a dose of thyroxine is being given to achieve the ideal therapeutic effect. Without being aware of these problems, the doctor is at risk of wrongly prescribing for his or her old patients, and this can be made more difficult by a person's own habit of self-prescribing. Sometimes large numbers of proprietary preparations are taken alongside the doctor's medicines. There is even a chance that old people are given drugs by friends and relatives that were originally prescribed for other people!

There is also the problem of whether old people take their prescribed treatment properly. Some do not understand the tablet-taking regime and, as a high proportion of old people are responsible for taking their own medicines, it is hardly surprising that many do not take their treatment as intended by the doctor. This is particularly true of patients living alone who are not receiving any regular supervision.

Under these circumstances, problems with adverse drug reactions are not uncommon. This has been highlighted by Professor James Williamson (1978), who carried out an investigation for the British Geriatrics Society into hospital admission at 42 geriatric departments. Of the admissions, 2.8% were necessitated solely by the adverse effects of drugs and 12.4% of the patients had adverse reactions of some kind. It appears that all doctors are faced with the problem, as Professor Williamson found that the level of adverse reactions amongst the patients being referred to geriatric wards from other departments in the hospital was the same as in patients being admitted from their homes.

It is of prime importance to make an accurate diagnosis. Only with this will effective treatment be possible. Difficulties arise, however, in old people because of the presence of several illnesses and these can often interact with each other. Some diseases are not amenable to treatment and some are perhaps better left alone. The doctor should have realistic aims when treating old people, and the effect of the drug given must be clear and have a purpose. This often means drawing up a system of priorities so that perhaps only the most important conditions and those most likely to respond are treated. A minimal number of drugs should be used and if larger quantities are necessary, they should be given for as short a time as possible. Other treatments, apart from pharmacological ones, are sometimes possible. Occasionally, changes in diet, attention to social difficulties and simple physiotherapy can be just as effective as drug treatment. The effect of arranging twice-weekly visits to luncheon centre can dramatically improve the outlook (and often the appetite) of a lonely old person. Oedema can disappear once mobility is restored. Above all, the reassuring presence of the doctor is often therapeutic.

The pharmacological action of the drugs used should be known to the doctor, who should be aware also of the correct doses for an old person and the possible side-effects and interactions of the drugs. It is useful to have regard to the body weight of the patient and adjust the dose accordingly, as in the case of children. The use of placebos and the purely symptomatic treatment of illness is sometimes necessary but this should be kept to a minimum and preferably used only for a limited period. Drugs that are likely to be beneficial should not be withheld just because a patient is old, but sometimes it is obvious that the effect of the drug on the patient is worse than the symptoms being treated, and it is better to cease treatment in these circumstances. In fact, it is sometimes more important and beneficial to take patients off treatment than to start new courses of tablets.

Many problems would be alleviated by adherence to the general principles of prescribing just outlined, but there are also organizational difficulties, an obvious one being the practice of repeat prescription. An old person on a drug needs reviewing at suitable intervals. Side-effects may arise that the patient him/herself will not report. Shaw and Opit (1976), studying the medication of 127 randomly selected patients aged over 70, found that about half the patients were on long-term treatment, 19 had no recorded contact with the family doctor for six months or longer, and examination by nurse surveillance suggested that 3 might be suffering from drug toxicity. They concluded that reliance on self-referral by elderly patients was unsafe. Periodic review of elderly patients on long-term treatment is therefore essential.

Drug compliance in elderly people can also be improved by education. Many devices have been recommended for improving patient under-standing of their medication. Instructions can be written down or trans-ferred on to a calendar. A tablet-identification card is helpful to augment written instructions. Supervisors can give the patient a daily supply in a small box and a check can be made later to see if they have been taken. Special packaging can be used with tablets marked for each day. Phar-macists can be helpful in giving specific and clear instructions to old patients and the habit of hoarding tablets could be reduced if the date of dispensing was noted on the label. A difficulty arises sometimes when patients are given tablets that have an unfamiliar appearance because they have been produced by a different drug manufacturer. The patient thinks this is a different drug and treats it with some suspicion and this is particularly true of patients discharged from hospital. The treatment of these patients needs to be carefully reviewed by the doctor and a check made that the patient is taking the tablets as instructed. The problem of approved names and proprietary names is also difficult for an old person to understand. A co-operation card held by the patient, showing the current treatment is useful in co-ordinating advice and therapy. The patient should be asked directly about any other medicines or pills that he/she is taking. Simplicity of treatment is essential; if one tablet can take the place of three, so much the better.

The White Paper *Working for Patients* includes proposals for indicative drug budgets for general practitioners. This would mean fixing the amount of money available to each GP for prescribing. If this results in more sensible prescribing and the introduction of personal or practice formularies it is to be welcomed. However from the point of view of elderly patients the increasing emphasis on anticipatory care is likely to increase the level of prescribing. Careful review of budgets will have to be made to take account of this and the likelihood of effective new products becoming available, which will extend therapeutic possibilities. To prepare realistic indicative drug budgets more information will need to be gathered about the morbidity pattern of each practice population.

ALTERNATIVE MEDICINE

Sometimes patients, including elderly people, use alternative or comple-mentary help, often with the knowledge and support of their doctor. The general attitude of the medical profession has changed considerably towards these alternatives and many doctors now practise some form of alternative medicine themselves, and others are ready to refer. This reflects a wider understanding and acceptance of the benefits of alternative forms of treatment. The range of possibilities is very wide. Old people most often use the services of an osteopath, a chiropractor, an acupuncturist and occasionally, a hypnotist. The contribution of other healers to the collective wellbeing of old people is welcome too. The effectiveness of their work should, however, be evaluated so that this contribution can be documented.

INVESTIGATIONS

Despite the fact that general practitioners tend not to undertake many investigations on old people, it is nevertheless an important possible outcome of a consultation and it is necessary to have an understanding of the interpretation of the investigations performed.

Biochemistry

There has been a considerable increase in the number of biochemical tests available during the past decade, and it is now usual to receive a comprehensive profile of such tests as a routine. It was initially impossible to find details of the normal range of these values for elderly people. These are now available in textbooks of geriatric medicine. Variations may occur in local pathological departments and their norms should be consulted where necessary. Most of the differences associated with old age in the normal values of biochemical tests, if they occur at all, are not usually of practical importance. Serum albumen tends to fall with age but not by very much (2–3 g per litre on the young-adult level). The only range that is markedly different in old age is that of serum phosphate, which falls considerably in old men so the appropriate range is lower than for young men and, indeed, for old women. The blood-urea level is not always indicative of renal function in elderly people. A substantial reduction of renal function can give normal blood urea.

Although old age itself has only minor effects, there are a number of other factors that influence the levels. These include illness itself, renal impairment, the effects of multiple pathology and disturbances due to drugs. When interpreting results, account has to be taken of any of these conditions which happen to be present. It is useful to inform the biochemist of coexistent factors and to discuss the results. Many of the effects produced by these conditions are complicated. Another problem is the way in which diseases present. Sometimes diseases presenting atypically only come to light as a result of wide-profile tests. Biochemical tests can, therefore, be used for screening, and interpretation becomes,

190 The old person in family medicine: clinical aspects

because of variations, difficult, and special care is needed. Consultation with the clinical pathologist is essential.

Haematology

The quantity and quality of the red and white cells do not change significantly with age. It has been suggested that erythrocyte sedimentation rate (ESR) increases with advancing age and that this is physiological. The range of normal values in old age is, however, uncertain. Perhaps a reason for this is the difficulty of identifying an unequivocably healthy elderly population. In a recent study of an age- and sex-matched sample of 200 subjects aged 60–89, Griffiths *et al.* (1984) have found that an ESR exceeding 19 mm per hour in men and 22 mm per hour in women warrants further investigation. Anaemia of any kind may result in an increase in ESR and this needs to be taken into account. Importantly, an ESR of 100 mm per hour or more is commonly associated with both giant-cell arteritis and polymyalgia rheumatica and this should be borne in mind.

The question arises as to what should be the normal level of haemoglobin in elderly people of both sexes. There have, however, been a wide range of values found in surveys of old persons, but it is suggested that figures of 13 g per dl for males and 12 g per dl for females are the lower ranges of normal haemoglobin levels.

Microbiology/virology

The most common bacteriological investigations undertaken in general practice in elderly people are on the urine. The incidence of bacteriuria increases with advancing age and is more common in females both young and old, but it is markedly more common in elderly males when compared with young males. Much of this bacteriuria is asymptomatic, although there are many causes for its presence. For a full discussion of this important subject a textbook of geriatric medicine should be consulted.

REFERENCES

Cartwright, A. and Smith, C. (1988) *Elderly People, their Medicines and their Doctors*, Routledge, London.
Griffiths, R.A., Good, W.R., Watson N.P., *et al.* (1984) Normal erythrocyte sedimentation rate in the elderly. *Br. Med. J.*, **289**, 724–5.
Illich, I. (1975) *Medical Nemesis. The exploration of health*, Marion Boyers, London.
Shaw, S.M. and Opit, L.J. (1976) Need for supervision of the elderly receiving long term prescribed medication. *Br. Med. J.*, **1**, 505–7.
WHO (1978) International Classification of Diseases (ninth revision), WHO, Geneva.

Wilkin, D., Metcalfe, D.H.M., Hallam, L. *et al.* (1984) Area variations in the process of care in urban general practice. *Br. Med. J.*, **289**, 229–32.

Wilkin, D., Hallam, L., Leavey, R. and Metcalfe, D. (1987) *Anatomy of Urban General Practice*, Tavistock, London.

Wilkin, D. and Williams, E.I. (1986) Patterns of care for the elderly in general practice. *J. R. Coll. Gen. Pract.*, **36**, 567–70.

Williams, E.I. (1983) The general practitioner and the disabled. *J. R. Coll. Gen. Pract.*, **33**, 296–9.

Williamson, J. (1978) Prescribing problems in the elderly. *Practitioner*, **220**, 749–55.

17 *The old person in family medicine*
Practice strategy

The community care of old people has become so important that it is necessary for all those who provide this care to work out their objectives and construct a programme through which these will be achieved. The problems presented by old people and the responses necessary to deal with these are universal and the strategy outlined in this chapter is relevant to any system of delivering primary medical care. The objectives of community care have been stated in Chapter 8, but when considering individual practice strategies, the guidelines suggested by Age Concern (1986) are very relevant. A summary of some of the most important suggestions follows. (The complete guidelines are available from Age Concern.)

GUIDELINES

Attitudes to patients and carers

Elderly patients can be clinically challenging in terms of diagnosis and treatment. It is often worth viewing older people in terms of their biological rather than their chronological status;

GPs, receptionists and medical secretaries need to ensure that they have a sympathetic attitude towards the needs of elderly people. This may require the provision of special training;

The primary health-care team should be responsive to the needs of minority groups including their cultural and religious practices;

Carers of elderly people must be given special attention;

Comprehensive information on the nature of the illness, its treatment and how it will progress should be provided to the patients unless it is judged not to be in their interest to have such details. This information, with the permission of the patient, needs to be provided to the carer;

Carers may need counselling on the risks that their elderly patients are taking;

Information on the range of services available to support carers or when to consult the doctor can usefully be provided in the form of practice booklets or information sheets.

Preventive care

Preventive work is an integral part of a comprehensive package;

Early identification and management of problems and, if necessary, referral to specialists, can often enable old people to enjoy better quality day-to-day lives;

Focused screening or case-finding techniques are preferable to screening entire elderly populations;

Most patients aged over 70 are seen at least once a year in the course of routine work. This is a good opportunity to conduct an annual check. Systems of reaching potential at-risk patients who are not in regular contact with a GP can then be established;

Screening of very simple and apparently minor complaints about which patients do not normally consult their doctor, for instance, relating to sight, hearing, feet and mobility, is very beneficial;

Preventive work can be undertaken within general-practice consultations or in special sessions for well elderly people.

Staff premises and organization

Anticipatory care is greatly facilitated by employing the full quota of ancillary staff and full use of attached staff;

Counsellors, chiropodists, physiotherapists, occupational therapists, dieticians and social workers could also be usefully employed as part of the team;

Patients should be allowed direct access to ancillary staff;

All members of the primary health-care team must have sufficient office accommodation and resources within the practice;

Close liaison with defined channels of communication and objectives and joint training may assist teamwork;

All practices should be accessible to disabled people and sited on ground floors. Where this is not so, help should be requested from the health and local authorities with FPC support. Toilet facilities should be provided;

Appointment systems and arrangements for seeing GPs should be as flexible as possible so that patients do not have to wait too long. It is important to recognize that many old people either do not have telephones or are reluctant to use them;

The needs of old people cannot always be met within the average short consultation, so additional time has to be allocated;

Age/sex registers are useful tools for identifying at-risk patients;

It may be helpful to keep a record of those patients who have not been seen in the course of a year so that a check can be made that they do not need help;

Consideration might be given to restructuring patients' records when they reach the age of 65. This restructuring should be accompanied by an up-to-date examination with some standard investigations.

Prescribing/home visits/GP-interest groups

It is good practice to monitor closely both patients' use of medicines (including self-medication) and any discernible trends in prescribing habits, perhaps by an annual review of the prescribed drugs. Methods to consider include prescription cards, drug sheets, repeat registers, patient prescription booklets and the use of computers;

Elderly patients can be helped to understand how to take their medicines by GPs issuing clear directions and advice to patients and carers, verbally and perhaps also written. The GP can work with the pharmacists and other members of the primary health-care team on methods of promoting compliance, encouraging the use of memory aids, keeping the number of different drugs taken in any one period to a minimum, monitoring at-risk patients, encouraging pharmacists to use easy-to-open bottles and large print on labels;

A careful balance between the need to encourage independence in the patient and the need to provide home visits should be struck;

Each request for a home visit should be carefully considered and not necessarily left to administrative staff to decide;

A home visit may be necessary if a patient is receiving complex treatment and is unfit to come to the surgery, has just recently been discharged from hospital, has been visited by a community nurse who indicates a GP visit is necessary, is recently bereaved, is in a home environment that requires review, or who has a carer who is experiencing problems;

Exchange of ideas can be achieved by GPs meeting in special-interest groups on a regular basis.

These principles are not only important to doctors but also to all members of the primary-care team. Patients and their carers also need to know how the service is organized and what it intends to achieve. The voice of the whole team and the consumers should be heard when planning practice strategies.

Many of the aspects to be considered when planning practice strategy have already been discussed in other parts of this book, but for convenience important points are summarized here.

**Summary of important points to be considered
when planning practice strategy**

Organization

The first thing to consider is the basic organizational framework providing care for elderly people. This involves having an age/sex register,
a disease or disability register and ideally an attendance register (see
Chapter 16). These can be computerized. The records should be reviewed
and contain problem lists, assessment details, drug information and properly filed letters and investigations. Details of the telephone number and
carer information about each patient is helpful. Practice organization in
terms of availability and accessibility to old people, especially appointment systems should be reviewed. Notes should be made of hospital
admission and discharge, often in central registers. The policy of not
accepting persons to the doctors' lists or in moving an old person already
on the list purely because of age is to be deplored. Careful policy discussions should be undertaken to make sure that this is avoided.

Acute care

Response to immediate problems is usually done well in family medicine.
Patients are usually seen at home in response to urgent calls for visits
within a short time and most patients manage to get appointments for
less urgent problems within a reasonable time. However, it is important
to review the arrangements for early appointments especially for old
persons.

Continuing care

There is a balance between providing too much follow-up care or too little.
Obviously there is no need to follow up every acute episode of illness in
old age. There are, however, some situations where maintenance or
regular follow-up arrangements need to be made. The routine visit was
often the way in which this was achieved, but with many patients having
access to transport, health-centre appointments are becoming more appropriate. If a patient is housefast, a visit is clearly necessary. Continuing
care is usually disability oriented. Patients who suffer from specific diseases, for example, stroke, diabetes, dementia, depression, incontinence,
heart failure, mobility problems, failing vision, etc., need to be seen
regularly, especially where there are difficulties in self-care. Sometimes
carers need support and regular contact. Patients on repeat prescriptions
need to have regular review. Using a computer helps to provide re-
minders of this. It is not always necessary for a doctor to undertake
continuing care. Health visitors and practice nurses can also effectively
provide this service.

Preventive care

Every primary-care group needs a policy on preventive care. The possibilities have been described in Chapters 10, 11 and 12. The need to make assessments at critical points, for instance, discharge from hospital, admission to residential accommodation, change in domestic circumstances, must be recognized and become part of care policy.

Role of the team

The role of the team in providing primary care for old persons is very important. The contribution of each member needs to be clarified and understood. The practice nurse or nurse practitioner should be available by direct access for old people and they should understand which services are given in the treatment room. Many practice nurses are now visiting old people at home. It is likely that a change in availability of practice ancillary workers will mean increased availability of nursing and counselling services in the practice. One such worker could be a link person who would liaise with hospital, social services, voluntary organizations, self-help groups and the geriatric-nursing liaison team. The important part played by receptionists and secretaries should be recognized. As first-line workers they set the scene for the care provided and are responsible for the necessary organizational backing. Education of all members of the team is important. Courses should be organized and members encouraged to attend.

Information

The attitude in primary care to providing information about services is changing rapidly. It used to be thought that distributing such information was bordering on advertising. Problems caused by this fear are now disappearing. Many practices supply leaflets that give details of the practice, the services that are offered and how to get them. These are available to all patients. This is a development that should help old people, and practices or groups should consider providing an information sheet or booklet.

Patient participation

Patient- or user-participation groups have been a feature of primary care in the United Kingdom for several years. They have not been widely adopted, but when they do exist, the most successful part is often concerned with elderly people. Not only do they function as a forum for discussion about problems in the service and ways of dealing with these, but also as a way of providing health education. The health centre becomes the location for regular meetings with invited speakers on a range of health topics. The voice of the consumer can be heard and thus responded to. Practical help can emerge from these groups in the form of help with transport and visiting services.

Carer programme

The problems faced by carers are detailed in Chapter 15. Relationships between the professionals and the prime carers need sensitive handling. Carers are usually spouses or members of the family and they are often patients of the practice themselves. The need for support is therefore doubly necessary. The need to balance the interests of patients and carers must be recognized. Problems of information sharing and confidentiality might arise, but in practice this is not a common occurrence.

Audit

Quality assessment has become an important recent development in primary care. Always a hallmark of professionalism, the need to monitor the service provided has now been widely accepted and in many instances formalized. Better health care through resultant clinical standard setting is likely and the proposals on audit included in the White Paper 'Working for Patients' are to be welcomed. Audit can take many forms. Monitoring the service means providing figures, for instance, about the consultation rate, the referral rate, the investigation rate, the visiting rate, etc. These are very useful as they allow a practice to compare itself with other practices and also for observing trends over time or identifying areas of deficiency. Audit itself is a more complicated activity and involves standard setting. It can apply to organizational procedures and clinical matters. The sequence is first, to identify a subject for audit, second to agree and define acceptable standards for the subject to be studied, third to undertake the audit review and finally, to compare what is found to be happening with the previously agreed acceptable standards. If there is a deficit, steps can then be taken to correct matters and a further evaluation undertaken later. The educational value of such an exercise is enormous. An example of organizational audit would be analysis of how long an old person has to wait to get an appointment. An example of a clinical audit would be how regularly elderly diabetics are seen for review and whether the patient has eye, feet and blood-sugar examinations undertaken on each review occasion.

FURTHER READING

Age Concern (1986) Meeting the needs for older people: some practice guidelines. September 1986. *Age Concern*, London.
Almind, G., Freer, C.B., Gray, J.A.M. and Warshaw, G. (Eds) (1983) The contribution of the primary care doctor to the medical care of the elderly in the community. *A Report from the Kellogg International Scholarship Program on Health*

and Aging (1983), the University of Michigan, USA.

Pritchard, P. (1981) (Ed.) *Patient participation in general practice.* Occasional Paper No 17. Royal College of General Practitioners, London.

Royal College of General Practitioners (1985) *Policy Statement no 2: Quality in general practice.* Royal College of General Practitioners, London.

Sheldon, M.G. (1982) *Medical Audit in General Practice.* Occasional Paper no 20. Royal College of General Practitioners, London.

Thompson, M.K. (1986) *Caring for an Elderly Relative. A guide to home care.* Martin Dunitz, London.

18 Nursing the elderly in the community

Traditionally, district nurses have been involved in providing a reactive service for elderly people, whereas health visitors have been involved in searching out health needs and providing an anticipatory service. The emphasis in district nursing has been placed firmly on direct care, but the distinction is slowly disappearing with district nurses becoming more involved in health education and the prevention of ill health.

Modern medicine relies absolutely on nursing help, both in the hospital and in the community. When dealing with a sick old person it is essential to involve the community nursing sister at as early a stage as possible in the illness so that as well as providing care and therapy, she can also prevent certain problems and complications from developing. Early contact also allows the nurse to form good relationships with patients and carers. In the last few years, particularly since the introduction of the new training syllabus for district nurses and the nursing process, the nurse has become involved in assessing the needs and problems of both patient and family. From this a nursing management plan is formulated, which incorporates medical treatment. The patient and carer are often included in this decision making. The aims of care are specified and regular evaluation takes place. As discussed in Chapter 8, community nurses generally work in teams consisting of a qualified district nurse who is supported by staff nurses without a district-nurse qualification, state-enrolled nurses and auxiliary nurses. Each patient receives care from an appropriate member of the team. In most, but not all areas, there is provision for patients to receive care outside normal hours. The nursing service has patients referred to it by general practitioners and also directly from the hospital.

Special difficulties are presented by nursing old people at home. They are often frail and suffer from multiple pathology. There may be mental impairment present so that instructions may not be fully understood. A task that could quite easily be carried out by younger patients may be beyond the ability of more elderly patients. Drugs may be forgotten and tablet taking may be quite haphazard and irregular. Old people may be lonely and cease caring for themselves. Nurses may be the only visitors to motivate them and their often ageing carers to attend to diet and hygiene.

In the community, nurses are called on to care for three types of situation. First, there is the acutely ill old person with, for instance, bronchitis.

This needs a full range of general nursing care, but usually only for a short limited time. Into this category also comes the post-operative patient discharged from hospital. The aim in caring for this type of patient is to restore the person to full health and a normal place in the community. Second, the nursing services may be involved in the long-term maintenance of, for instance, the patient who has had a stroke or is suffering from multiple sclerosis. Here the patient may be ambulant, but nevertheless requires some nursing care to supervise continuing rehabilitation, incontinence and healing pressure sores. Supervision of a diabetic patient at home would come into this category. Third, there is the nursing of the bedfast patient at home. This usually means terminal care.

BASIC PRINCIPLES OF NURSING A PATIENT AT HOME

As has been mentioned it is essential for the nurse to arrive early on the scene. Nurses should educate their doctors to alert them at the beginning of an illness and not to leave it until it is obvious to all that nursing care is imperative. The room where the patient is to be nursed needs to be adequately heated and lighted. It is sometimes more convenient to nurse an ill old patient downstairs than in a cramped bedroom. This may also be easier for the family and facilitate earlier rehabilitation. At home the bed is often too low – but it can be raised with blocks. It must be at a height that is safe for the patient to get in and out of. Ideally when the patient sits on the edge of the bed the feet should be flat on the floor. Occasionally, safety sides are necessary when there is a danger of the patient falling out of bed. It is possible to obtain hospital beds with sides for use in the home and these should be installed, as makeshift arrangements are seldom satisfactory. A bed table is also helpful, especially the cantilever type with adjustable height and angle. Bedding needs to be light and warm. Linen is not provided but some health authorities have laundry services that collect soiled linen and return it laundered to the patient's home. Some people prefer duvets, but they can be difficult to keep clean. Sheepskins are available and many find them very comfortable. Old people slip down the bed easily and at home, ingenious relatives have sometimes been able to fix overhead handles for the patient to clasp. A rope ladder attached to the end of the bed can also help in some situations. In general old people should be encouraged to stay in bed for as little time as possible. This minimizing of bed rest is a fundamental precept of nursing at home. As the patient recovers, the relatives will need instructing as to how best to get the patient in and out of bed. There are special gadgets, such as hoists, available for moving a very disabled patient at home, although hospital admission may be necessary when this is difficult. Usually a patient can be helped to swing his/her legs over the side of the bed until he/she is sitting upright. After a pause, he/she should be able to stand. The patient will also need help with dressing and undressing at this stage.

Dehydration can occur all too easily in elderly people and adequate fluid intake is necessary. The diet also needs supervising with special care to ensure that sufficient vitamins are taken. Toileting arrangements are important and the nurse may well have to resort to certain aids such as the use of a commode so that toileting is easy and comfortable. General attention to personal care such as washing, bathing, shaving and hair-brushing is necessary. This helps the patient to preserve his or her self-respect. It is important that old people are treated as individuals; for instance, if possible, bed bathing should be kept to a minimum and they should be encouraged to wash themselves and allowed to use their own bath or shower. Clothes, too, should be kept clean and changed frequently. Community nurses are also involved in some very useful preventive work. This includes the avoidance of pressure sores, minimizing the effect of both urinary and faecal incontinence and avoiding contractures.

Community nurses have a very special responsibility in supervising treatment. Tablets need to be taken regularly and watch kept for side-effects. This is much more difficult at home than in the hospital where there is the traditional drug round and total nursing supervision for the whole twenty-four hours of the day. At home this is impractical and the nurse has to rely on members of the family or neighbours to undertake general supervision. This involves her in the task of educating these helpers in what needs to be done and how to recognize relevant improvement or deterioration. If these extra helpers are not available when a patient lives alone, night sitting and home-help services may be possible, but if not, it is sometimes better for the patient to be admitted to hospital. The part played by district nurses in co-ordinating other services is, however, very important in avoiding such admissions.

In the community the nurse might find herself very much concerned with other tasks apart from straightforward nursing. She may well be asked to undertake simple physiotherapy, including training a patient to use aids. Occupational and speech therapy may also be necessary, particularly for those suffering from stroke. This general rehabilitation role of the community sister is very important and can be the critical factor that leads the patient successfully through acute illness back to independence.

Very often an old person's perception of the environment is retained even when bedfast, and recovery may be helped by bright and cheerful surroundings as well as the general encouragement of those giving nursing care. Some may become very dependent on the nurse and this applies even more so in the community than in hospital. The dilemma sometimes exists as to how firm to be in insisting that certain tasks should be undertaken by patients themselves and how much to do for them because of their disability. It is very easy to do more than is necessary in order to save time. The hospital geriatric-liaison nursing team can often help if this is a problem.

The social services department will provide aids and appliances to make nursing at home easier. These include chemical toilets, commodes, tripods, Zimmer frames, monkey chains to make moving up the bed easier, high chairs, bath seats, handrails and ramps. A community occupational therapist will be helpful in discussing the needs of an elderly person for such aids. The community nursing services will provide equipment for the comfort of the patient in bed, including disposable sheets and pads. Incontinence aids for those suffering from incontinence are also provided. In general, the social services departments provide aids to living and the nursing services provide aids to nursing, but there is some overlap. The Marie Curie Foundation makes allowances to patients suffering from cancer for extra diet and other comforts and is also very helpful in providing night sitters.

Communication is helped by nursing records being left at the patient's home. Temperature charts are unnecessary, but notes made of temperature and pulse in acutely ill patients are useful. The doctor should also record changes in medical treatment. Messages can be left on the record sheets, but there is no real substitute for direct verbal communication between doctor and nurse.

Geriatric community-nursing teams are available in some areas. They co-ordinate discharge into the community and offer support and advice to relatives. Their duties are to liaise with hospital medical, nursing and social staff and their counterparts in the community. They also make special visits to those on the waiting list for admission to hospital. Supervision of continuing rehabilitation of discharged hospital patients may also be part of their duties.

The practice nurse usually works from the surgery and ideally has a treatment room at her disposal so that she can treat ambulant old people. The range of care might include giving injections, dressing ulcers and dealing with injuries. General supervision of treatment may also be undertaken for patients with hypertension or diabetes. An old person may be referred for specific treatment such as ear syringing or for treating eye infections.

There are four different areas in which nursing care is very important in the community. These are the management of pressure sores, incontinence, contractures and restless patients. These will be described briefly here.

Pressure sores

Pressure sores can be either superficial or deep. Superficial sores are usually due to small injuries of the skin caused by sheering forces and friction as a result of moving a patient up the bed. They are the most common form of ulcer and may account for up to 90% of the total. They may become infected and this is particularly liable to occur where urinary incontinence is also present. Deep sores, which are sometimes called decubitas ulcers, are more serious and occur when the skin over a bony prominence is compressed for any length of time. This causes the blood supply to be cut off with resulting tissue destruction. This may occur without the skin surface actually being broken, and discolouration may not appear immediately. Nevertheless, extensive damage may have occurred to the underlying tissues. Areas particularly vulnerable to developing this type of sore are over the main bony prominences such as the pelvis, the buttocks and the lower part of the back. They can occur over the shoulder blades and elbows. The resultant sore is usually deep and can sometimes be covered by a hard scab that hides the necrotic changes that have taken place underneath. Other factors also contribute to the development of ulcers. Incontinence can cause skin sogginess. Unconscious and paralysed patients are vulnerable as well as those who are thin and emaciated. Arteriosclerosis can reduce the blood supply to the skin and make ulceration more likely. Fever, dehydration and poor nutrition may also be contributory. The use of a hot-water bottle may sometimes cause a burn that may become infected and ulcerated. Nurses assess the risk of pressure sores forming with a 'Norton score' by considering the patient's physical and mental activity, morbidity and incontinence status. These are individually scored from 1 to 4 and patients with a total score of 14 or less are liable to develop sores (Norton, McLaren and Exton-Smith, 1962).

Prevention of sores
Bed sores, both superficial and deep, are in many ways a tragic occurrence and as they are difficult to treat, prevention is of prime importance when nursing old people. Damage can often be done in the first week of illness, or even overnight, and therefore prevention should be instituted early. The position of an old person should be changed as frequently as possible and the period of bed rest reduced to a minimum. The change in position may have to be as often as every two hours in an unconscious paralysed patient. The movement also helps to prevent chest infection. Sheepskins are regularly used and there are specially shaped ones to protect heels and ankles. There may be a danger of developing a pressure sore on the buttock if the patient is sat out of bed too soon and remains immobile in a chair. Special care should be taken to keep the skin clean. Soap and water is probably the best way of cleaning the skin. The traditional methylated spirits and powder applications are now no longer advocated. Barrier creams such as Vasogen (Pharmax) and Conotrane (WBP) may be used to protect vulnerable areas. This can also be achieved

conveniently by using an aerosol spray of which Sprilon (Pharmax) is a popular example, especially when there is early reddening, although it is expensive to use continually. Opsite (S & N) spray is often used for superficial sores and is very effective. The general condition of the patient needs attention with a special watch kept for dehydration. A diet rich in protein and with added vitamins is helpful. If incontinence is a problem, an indwelling catheter may become necessary. Sedation should be avoided so that the patient is capable of moving naturally. Attention should also be paid to the skin areas that are vulnerable, especially for early changes in colour. Heel sores can develop when the patient finds it difficult to move his/her legs because of tight sheets, and a cradle may prevent this.

Many special mattresses have been developed to help in the prevention of sores and are considerably more sophisticated than the original sheepskins. Few, however, are of much value in the home. Ripple or alternative-pressure mattresses can be used, but although they might save nurses' time they do need careful supervision and a reliable electricity supply. New technical developments are producing beds that may eventually solve the problem, ranging from hammock types to a continuously inflated air mattress. They are expensive and it will possibly be a long time before they are seen in the patient's home.

Treatment

Superficial sores should be cleaned with soap and water or a non-irritant lotion such as Cetrimide 1% and after being allowed to dry, sprayed with Sprilon or Opsite. Healing usually takes place slowly, although sometimes infection may be present and then a swab should to taken for bacteriological assessment. However, antibiotics are not usually necessary.

Deep sores need to be cleaned and necrotic tissue removed. This can usually be done using forceps and scissors but powders are available such as Debrisan (Pharmax) to soften the slough. Sometimes it is helpful to dissolve the powder in a little glycerine. Debrisan is expensive and cheaper products include Aserbine (Bencard) and Malatex (Norton). Surgical treatment is rarely needed in old age, but if the ulcer is extensive and the patient's condition is good, surgical advice about the possibility of grafting may be justified.

Urinary incontinence

In recent years a much deeper understanding has been gained of the causes of urinary incontinence, which has led to improvement in management. A full account of the changes associated with ageing and the anatomical and physiological background to the mechanisms can be found in textbooks of geriatric medicine. From the practical point of view, however, incontinence may be due to diseases of the brain or spinal cord (neuropathic) or local abnormalities in the bladder and urinary tract (focal). These produce different types of bladder abnormality. Cases of neuropathic urinary incontinence characteristically have a hypersensitive bladder that empties frequently without the patient being aware of this taking place. The bladder is not usually palpable as its capacity is reduced and it is small and contracted. On the other hand, focal lesions, which interfere with the emptying, are usually associated with a full bladder and overflow incontinence. The patient wets him/herself but on examination, a full bladder is found. Causes can include such things as urethral caruncle, urinary infection and prolapse in the female, and prostatic hypertrophy in the male. Constipation may be a cause in both. Associated with these are overlying emotional and environmental problems. It sometimes happens that a patient in an acute period of stress may be incontinent but once this has passed, full continence returns. Some environmental changes, such as going to hospital or sleeping in a strange bed, can precipitate incontinence, often with great embarrassment to the old person. Severe illness of any sort can produce incontinence. Diabetes mellitus may be an associated finding. Because of increased frequency and reduced bladder capacity in old age, immobility is a potent background cause of incontinence. This may, for instance, occur after an operation.

Nursing management in the first place means assessment to establish the cause and decide on the best way to alleviate the problem. This means determining the type of incontinence, its frequency and pattern and also any precipitating causes. The patient's mental and mobility state also need to be assessed. Close co-operation between the doctor and nurse is very important at this stage. Treatment of any cause found should be instituted. For instance if there is a local lesion present, help from a urological or gynaecological surgeon may be necessary. Rectal examination may reveal faecal impaction, which is causing the condition. Sometimes chronic constipation needs to be treated. Infections, if present, should be remedied, and bacterial examination of the urine is necessary to determine causal bacteria. Glycosuria should also be excluded. Sometimes a full urological examination may be necessary, including intravenous pyelography and cystoscopy.

It may prove impossible to control the incontinence by formal treatment and this is when nursing management becomes important. There is little joy in dealing with an incontinent old patient and it may be tempting to show distaste and annoyance at the continual unclean and wet state. Some old people even give the impression that they are incontinent on purpose as an attention-seeking device. This is rarely the case and much can be achieved by understanding the problem and urging the patient to keep as active as possible. In the first place, therefore, the patient should be treated sympathetically and with general reassurance, remembering that they are often extremely embarrassed by their problem. Aids to mobility, regular toileting and an alarm clock to act as a reminder may be all that is necessary. The bladder should always be emptied before retiring. It is helpful to make sure that the patient has adequate recourse to a bedside commode or bottle, particularly at night. Sedatives are best kept to a minimum and restriction of fluid in the evening may be valuable for patients suffering from nocturnal incontinence. Diuretics sometimes produce incontinence and careful timing of the dosage is important.

There are a number of drugs used in the treatment of incontinence. Anticholinergic drugs permit increased relaxation of the bladder and an increased volume. The side effects are retention of urine, blurring of vision and dryness of the mouth. It is helpful if an incontinence chart is kept so that the pattern of micturition can be anticipated and the drugs prescribed accordingly: the dosage may need to be changed. It there is no progress, the treatment would have to be discontinued. When depression is present incontinence may be helped by antidepressant drugs.

Despite these measures the condition is often persistent and recourse has to be made to incontinence aids. Disposable incontinence pads are very useful for the patient in bed and they can absorb up to 300 ml of urine. The person should sit directly on them without intervening clothes. For this reason they are not suitable for use when patients are sitting in a chair. Disposable napkins or pants are available and a variety very popular with patients are Kanga pants. They ingeniously hold the pad in a waterproof pouch outside the pants which are made of one-way water-repellent fabric that allows the urine through into the disposable pad. About 400 ml of urine can be held and there is no need to remove the pants to change the pad. Some local authorities arrange for the disposable pads to be collected from the house at intervals. In the male, penile clamps or condom drainage is sometimes helpful. Special care of the skin and scrupulous hygiene is always needed in these cases. Permanent catheterization is sometimes necessary. The plastic balloon catheter is the one usually used. The balloon is usually filled with sterile water using a 20 ml syringe. Infection is always the risk with this type of catheter and even with an inflated balloon, patients can sometimes pull it out. Noxyflex solution (Geistlich) should be instilled into the bladder if infection is present, either weekly or an alternate days. Long-term antibiotic therapy is not used routinely with elderly patients. Foley's balloon catheter needs changing monthly but the Silastic or Dover's catheters need only to be changed every three months and are a great improvement. Although always a difficult task, nursing this type of patient at home is now much more feasible because of the new improved catheters. Carers and relatives need considerable support when nursing incontinence patients. Tolerance of the problem is low and full explanation and help is needed. Extra laundry can produce a financial burden and attendance allowance should be applied for. In some areas a nursing adviser on incontinence is available.

Faecal incontinence

This is a distressing condition that often occurs in bedfast demented patients. It is commonly due to faecal compaction and produces spurious diarrhoea. Neoplasm of the bowel is another possible cause. Short-term incontinence may be associated with an attack of diarrhoea caused by infection of the bowel or dietary disturbance. Any serious illness may be associated with faecal incontinence and some drugs such as antibiotics and iron may cause diarrhoea in an old person and precipitate incontinence. Self-prescribed large doses of laxatives are not uncommon in elderly people and may produce diarrhoea. Nursing treatment involves attention to any predisposing causes and relief of the impaction if present. This usually involves enemas or rectal washout and sometimes manual removal. Suppositories, for instance glycerine, may be helpful. It may also be useful to increase the volume of faeces by using a high-residue diet containing bran. Certain foods cause diarrhoea in some patients and if these can be recognized, they should be avoided. If diarrhoea is persistent once infection or neoplasm have been excluded, Kaolin mixture may help to harden the stools. General attention to training and suitable clothing should be instituted as outlined in the section on urinary incontinence. Faecal incontinence is usually preventable and reversible. Diet and fluid are important, so are privacy, comfort and time to promote normal defecation.

Avoiding contractures

When nursing a bedfast or partially bedfast old person, it is important to realize how easily contractures may develop. A stroke patient may be discharged back home and without careful supervision may very quickly develop a contracture. They are usually associated with prolonged stay in bed and when this is inevitable, active and passive movements of the limbs that are at risk should be encouraged. If the joints are painful, analgesics should be given to allow them to move more freely. Bedclothes should not be pulled tightly around the legs as restriction of movement can sometimes cause knee-stiffening or foot-drop.

Nursing a restless patient

There are many causes of restlessness in an old person. Infections, particularly pneumonia, or any acute illness, and also such conditions as heart failure and anaemia may make an old person sleepless. Impairment of consciousness often associated with brain failure and developing cerebral thrombosis can aggravate the condition. Uraemic patients may be particularly fretful and disoriented at night. Certain drugs used in sedation may give rise to agitation and this is particularly true of bromides and barbiturates. Other drugs may also be responsible and therapy should be reviewed when restlessness is present. Pain and discomfort may contribute and may result from a full bladder or faecal impaction. Old persons who will not settle at night are well known to nurses. They may be reasonably co-operative through the day, but once the evening arrives, they may wander around noisily, upsetting everyone by their disorientation. Tranquillizers are helpful and the most usual ones used are Sparine and Largactil, both in syrup form. General measures, such as keeping the patient up during the day and ensuring some activity, not going to bed too soon, and providing a bedtime milky drink may, however, be all that is necessary.

CONCLUSION

Nursing elderly people at home is a task that demands the full resources of nursing skill. There are special difficulties involved and this demands understanding on the part of the community nursing team to achieve success. Apart from nursing, the tasks undertaken by the community team involve rehabilitation, patient education, attention to diet and keeping an eye on the general social state of the patient. Supporting relatives and carers is an important part of the nurse's role and this may continue after a bereavement.

FURTHER READING

Kratz, C.R. (1978) *The Care of the Long-term Sick in the Community*, Churchill Livingstone, Edinburgh and London.
Mandelstam, D. (1977) *Incontinence: a Guide to the Understanding of a very Common Complaint*, Heineman Medical Books, London.
Norton, C. (1986) *Nursing for Continence*, University Press, Oxford.
Norton, D., McLaren, R. and Exton-Smith, A.N. (1962) *An Investigation of Geriatric Nursing Problems in Hospital*, Churchill Livingstone, Edinburgh.

19 Common problems in family medicine

INTRODUCTION

It is necessary in family medicine, when dealing with elderly people, to widen the concept of diagnosis. Multiple pathology is the rule in old age and in terms of diseases present, several diagnoses are possible at any given time. Often these are quite separate in themselves and involve different systems. Their treatment is usually distinct. However, they must also be considered collectively because several different pathologies can produce a cumulative effect on function and relatively minor conditions often together produce a significant problem. Thus a bunion associated with mild osteoarthritis of a hip joint can, especially in an overweight patient, seriously reduce mobility. The 'diagnosis' would be an osteoarthritic hip in a person who was overweight with a bunion on the right foot who had, as a result of these three conditions, significant loss of mobility. This more fully describes the problem. The importance of loss of function makes it necessary to make a diagnosis, not only in terms of diseases present but also of the effect these have on function.

It is therefore impossible to consider individual diseases as separate entities when caring for elderly persons (Thompson, 1986). The principle of defining problems in *functional* terms and then seeking solutions to them in these terms is very important. The solutions are very often non-pharmacological and can include physiotherapy and various social inputs. This book is not concerned with the description of the diseases of old age – there are many excellent textbooks available that do this – but there are certain conditions that occur in the community that contribute significantly to functional impairment. Included in this group are stroke, diabetes mellitus, certain mental disorders, acute confusion, vision and hearing defects and arthritis. In some specific diseases there is becoming an increasing tendency to construct protocols for their management in the community. This is an encouraging and helpful development.

STROKE

Stroke is a common condition and is the main cause of death in the UK after heart disease and cancer. Each year nearly two in every thousand of the population will suffer from stroke. Amongst elderly people, the incidence rises steeply. Strokes are responsible for considerable residual disability. In the community it is important that prompt initial care should be given and that this should be followed by effective continuing care.

The term 'stroke' is perhaps loosely applied to describe the clinical manifestation of two distinct happenings in the cerebrovascular system. These are sometimes referred to jointly as 'cerebrovascular accidents' (CVA). These are a haemorrhage or a blockage; the latter is usually by a clot or thrombus, but also by an embolus arising in the heart, or in the carotid or vertebral arteries. This blockage produces death of part of the brain supplied by the artery affected. The area of destroyed tissue is called an infarction. Thus cerebral thrombosis or occlusion produces cerebral infarction. The position and extent of the infarction determines the differing clinical pictures. Haemorrhage from a cerebral artery causes infusion of blood into the surrounding brain tissue and causes damage in this way, as well as by cutting off or reducing the blood supply to the parts supplied by the artery.

Within the group of cerebrovascular incidents are episodes of so-called transient ischaemic attacks (TIAs). The underlying cause is different and consists of a reduction in the blood supply to the brain that is only of short duration. This is due to temporary blockage of parts of the cerebral circulation by micro-emboli of dislodged platelets arising from atheromatous plaques situated at the bifurcation of the common carotid artery, the vertebro-basilar artery, or in some cases, the heart itself. The dislodgement of these emboli may be precipitated by a fall in the blood pressure from such causes as coronary thrombosis. Anaemia, hypoglycaemia and renal and hepatic failure can also help to cause transient ischaemic attacks. Obstruction of the blood supply to the brain by cervical spondylosis may also be contributory.

Transient ischaemic attacks

These are important as they may herald a full cerebral thrombosis. They are treatable and it may be possible to take action to avoid more serious trouble. The clinical findings can vary and depend on the source of the micro-emboli. Those arising in the carotid artery may be associated with eye symptoms such as hemianopia or even complete blindness, and also with limb weakness, which is usually unilateral. Speech defects may also occur. Sometimes a murmur may be audible over the carotid artery. When the source of the micro-emboli is the vertebro-basilar arterial system, the symptoms include dizziness, eye symptoms such as double vision, or sometimes complete loss of sight, limb weakness (which is often bilateral) and speech difficulty. Memory disturbances may also be a feature. Vertebro-basilar attacks are said to have a better prognosis and rarely proceed to full stroke. In practice, however, it is clinically often difficult to separate these two types. A careful examination of the heart may reveal disease, which may be the source of micro-embolism from this organ. Full recovery, however, takes place within a few minutes and certainly within twenty-four hours, although the attacks may be recurrent.

The clinical presentation of complete stroke can be very complex and the effects can range widely from the severe to the mild. Early symptoms of headache, unsteadiness and sensations of weakness can be experienced by the patient. These can often be remembered clearly and described dramatically at a later period. In the acute stage, consciousness may be lost and deep coma may ensue; in other cases the patient may remain lucid throughout the episode. A whole range of neurological deficits can occur, but most commonly the person is left with a hemiplegia, together with weakness of the facial muscles and sometimes a speech defect. Other conditions may be present at the same time as a stroke and some, such as hypertension or a fibrillating heart, may have led directly to the attack. It is often impossible to distinguish clearly between cerebral thrombosis and cerebral haemorrhage; the latter is most likely to be the underlying event if there is a pre-existing hypertension and is more likely to occur in a younger individual. In both haemorrhage and embolus, the onset of stroke is likely to be sudden.

Treatment of transient ischaemic attacks usually involves two or three days of rest and a gradual resumption of activity within a week. Any possible underlying cause such as anaemia, drug misuse or hypoglycaemia should be treated and this would mean doing investigations such as full blood count, blood-sugar level, chest X-ray and ECG. Temporal arteritis is sometimes a cause of transient ischaemic attack and ESR or blood viscosity should be done to check for this. Serological studies can be included in the investigations to exclude rare cases of neurosyphilis. Blood pressure should be monitored and the diastolic level kept below 100 mm Hg by using antihypertensive agents if necessary. There are arguments in favour of full hospital investigation of patients who have suffered from transient ischaemic attacks because it may be possible to prevent further episodes and particularly the onset of a full cerebral accident by surgical procedures such as endarterectomy. The question of anticoagulation on a long-term basis will have to be considered. In very elderly patients, careful thought needs to be taken as to whether this is worthwhile.

In recent years drugs such as aspirin and dipyridamole (Persantin) have been used to modify platelet function. The hope is that these drugs will inhibit platelet aggregation and thus prevent the adherence of platelets in an area of damaged endothelium. Dipyridamole is sometimes used in combination with aspirin or can be used alone. Side effects do occur and it is necessary to be cautious because the drug may exacerbate migraine and hypotension. There has been some uncertainty about the dose of aspirin but a British Medical Journal Leading Article in January 1988 (Orme, 1988) comes down firmly with the recommendation of 300 mg daily. It would seem advisable to use an enteric-coated preparation of aspirin. If there is any doubt about the nature of the transient ischaemic attack and its underlying cause, it is always helpful to get the advice of a consultant geriatrician so that the situation can be fully explored.

The management of stroke

Several immediate actions may be needed when faced with a person suffering from a full cerebrovascular accident. Urgent first aid is often necessary and breathing difficulty may make it essential to ensure a clear airway. False teeth should be removed and the inhalation of vomit avoided by positioning the patient on his/her side. There is usually little doubt as to the diagnosis but if the doctor is early on the scene there may be difficulty in deciding whether someone has suffered from a full stroke or merely a transient ischaemic attack. Sometimes the problem is solved by rapid improvement of symptoms but in any event if the general condition of the patient is satisfactory, the doctor can reasonably wait a little before making a final diagnosis. Sometimes cases present with increased intra-cranial pressure as demonstrated by the presence of papilloedema. Other conditions apart from cerebrovascular accident may produce raised pressure and the doctor should enquire for a history of injury and consider the possibility of a resulting subdural haematoma. A history of headache, especially in the presence of papilloedema, may indicate the presence of cerebral tumour. Infection may also produce a similar clinical picture and a note should be taken of a raised temperature and neck stiffness to exclude the presence of, for instance, meningitis. Many other conditions can also mimic cerebrovascular accident in old age and these can include epilepsy, migraine, cardiac conditions, Stokes–Adams attacks and hypoglycaemia.

All these possibilities should be borne in mind by the doctor when making an initial assessment, but following this, it will be necessary to make the often difficult decision as to whether to admit the patient to hospital. In cases of transient ischaemic attacks, most GPs would be prepared to treat the condition at home, but with complete stroke, the decision is not as clear. Some will say that all stroke patients should be admitted to hospital and although this may be theoretically correct, there are others who are prepared to treat mild cases at home. There are several factors to be considered. The patient's clinical condition is often all-important. Mild hemiplegias with rapidly recovering movement may be suitable for home care. Sometimes in the case of a very old patient, where detailed investigation is contra-indicated, it is better to keep him/her at home and thus avoid the stresses, both mental and physical, of being transferred by ambulance to the new environment of a hospital. Extension of a stroke can indeed sometimes be precipitated by such movement. If death is imminent and the condition is obviously terminal, it is more humane to nurse the patient at home and hospital admission should be avoided.

The nature and extent of extracerebral disease also needs assessing and when such conditions as heart failure and bronchopneumonia concurrently present, this will indicate hospital admission. A previous history of stroke may mean transfer, as also is the case when there is impaired consciousness. If the general health of the patient was good before the stroke and there is no hypertension, it is reasonable to consider home management.

Another important consideration is whether adequate nursing is available. Will the relatives be able to look after the patient and are there suitable bedroom facilities? Family reaction to strokes can vary; some insist that the patient be admitted to hospital and some insist on the reverse. Hospital admission becomes essential, however, when constant and complex treatment is likely to be necessary. Doubt may sometimes exist as to whether the condition is due to thrombosis or to treatable haemorrhage. In these cases, full investigation is indicated, including the examination of the cerebrovascular fluid and, if available, a CT scan. Neurosurgical treatment is available for cerebrovascular episodes due to haemorrhage and this is of course the argument for hospital admission of all stroke cases, so that full investigations can be carried out. This really is more important for younger subjects suffering from stroke caused by a possible subarachnoid haemorrhage. This is a special type of brain haemorrhage that may be helped surgically. In elderly people, however, the possibility of such neurosurgical intervention occurs much less frequently. There are regional variations in the facilities for investigation and only certain areas have special stroke units. When these are available, a fine balance of judgement is necessary when considering the question of whether to admit an old person to hospital or to proceed with home care.

Management of a case of completed stroke at home involves three things: medical care, nursing care and rehabilitation. Anticoagulants are obviously contraindicated at home but the use of steroids and diuretics as cerebral decongestants must be considered. There is also the problem as to whether to treat hypertension. The patient may be already on treatment and this should be continued. In the early stage of the stroke, it is probably unwise to reduce a raised blood pressure, but later, if the diastolic level is over 120 mm Hg, it may be necessary to use hypotensive or diuretic agents. The cardiac and renal state must be carefully assessed before embarking on this treatment. Generally in old age, hypotensive drugs should be used cautiously, particularly in established cerebro-vascular disease. The presence of dementia contraindicates their use completely.

Nursing care will involve the usual attention to such things as general washing, cleaning, toileting, maintenance of adequate fluid levels and dietary advice. Lifting paralysed patients up and down the bed requires care to avoid shoulder subluxation and is usually a two-handed task. The head should be elevated to reduce cerebral oedema. The period of bed rest should be reduced to as short a time as possible in order to reduce the risk of thrombosis in the veins of the calf muscles, hypostatic pneumonia, joint contractures and pressure sores.

Rehabilitation is vitally necessary if the patient is to make a good functional recovery and should start at the beginning of the illness. The stages of rehabilitation have been described elsewhere. It might be that physiotherapy fails to influence the neurological outcome but neverthe-less, the patient's ability to cope with daily living can probably be improved by exercises that improve general fitness and enable other working muscles to compensate. The success of this type of rehabilitation may be better at home than in hospital.

Continuing care

When the acute state has passed and life is preserved, the aim of manage-ment must be not only to enable the patient to make as full a functional recovery as possible, but also to avoid a recurrence of further strokes. This latter will probably mean investigations on the lines suggested for transient ischaemic attacks. Full recovery cannot, however, be expected in all cases of stroke and finally, the health-care team is left with pati-ents in whom residual damage is present, who were either managed at home in the first place or have been discharged from hospital. The full resources of rehabilitation services are necessary to enable this type of patient to adjust to the disability and the inevitability of a restricted life style. The patient's psychological adjustment to this situation also needs attention and the family's attitude to this needs to be discussed, particu-larly as this may involve considerable social adaptation. Help from all members of the primary health-care team should be forthcoming, par-ticularly to reassure the patient that he/she has not been forgotten once the initial episode has been successfully overcome. There are many severely handicapped hemiplegics who have benefited from successful rehabilitation in the early stages, but who regress once this is finally withdrawn. Support for the family under these circumstances is of vital importance because they are eventually left with most of the responsi-bility and they continue to need help, particularly when speech has been affected and communication with a patient is difficult. Home visits by members of the primary health-care team are very important in this sense. Voluntary organizations such as Age Concern and appropriate self-help groups can also be extremely helpful in these circumstances. Sometimes adaptations are needed to the house to enable the patient to move about more effectively. There is also a wide range of aids available and help from a social worker is often very valuable. Wheelchairs are also a very important help. An application should also be made for attendance allowance.

Finally, how possible is it to prevent stroke or recurrence of stroke in elderly people? This is uncertain but some precursor conditions such as diabetes, obesity and heart failure can be treated effectively and should be identified. There is the difficult problem of a raised blood pressure. No definitive evidence exists about the value of treating this in elderly people, but levels of diastolic pressure of over 105 mm Hg should make one consider the possibility. The place of long-term anticoagulants and arterial surgery in old age remain, however, still speculative. The use of aspirin, however, is becoming more common.

DIABETES MELLITUS

Elderly diabetic patients may be long-established, or have recently acquired the disease in its late-onset form. The prevalence of diabetes in old age is difficult to ascertain, partly because of the differing significance attached by experts to various levels of blood sugar in elderly patients. It is generally agreed that a fasting blood sugar of over 130 mg per 100 ml (7.2 mmol/litre) or a blood-sugar level, two hours after 50 mg of glucose by mouth has been administered, of over 200 mg per 100 ml (11.1 mmol/litre) indicates diabetes and the patient should be treated accordingly. For people with lower degrees of elevation it has been suggested that the treatment might be beneficial in reducing the specific complications of diabetes and also the frequency of arterial disease.

Up to a quarter of the population of patients over 75 years old have abnormal glucose-tolerance tests, but many of these patients are without glycosuria. Diabetes mellitus has been shown to be an undiagnosed condition in elderly people and in a survey of patients of over 75 years old in general practice, the prevalence of diabetes mellitus was 5%, of which half was previously unreported (Williams *et al.*, 1972).

The classical symptoms of thirst and polyuria are relatively uncommon in elderly people, although weight loss and pruritis may give the first hint of developing diabetes. Pruritis vulvae and balanitis are often present. A patient developing incontinence or bed-wetting should be suspected of the condition and again these are often early symptoms. Diabetes may also present as one of its complications. These include vascular disease due to arteriosclerosis either as coronary thrombosis or ischaemic disease of the lower limb. This latter, when combined with diabetic neuropathy, which often causes loss of sensation in the feet, can cause infected ulcers and eventually gangrene and is a serious complication. Old persons with a predisposition to infection should be suspected of having diabetes. Another complication that sometimes presents is renal failure. Keto-acidosis is rare in old people but any confused or comatose elderly patient should be suspected of having the disease, particularly if dehydrated. Abdominal pain may be a striking feature of diabetes in old age and often develops in people not previously known to be diabetic. A mild case of late-onset diabetes is sometimes found at a preventive screening clinic for elderly people by the finding of glycosuria. In these cases, estimation of the blood-sugar level is necessary for diagnosis. Most clinics do routine blood-sugar estimations and this is useful because a raised blood sugar may not be associated with glycosuria. Indeed the screening test for diabetes is a post-prandial blood-sugar estimation. Late-onset cases are usually mild and the complications are more important than the actual disease.

The problem facing the doctor once a diagnosis of late-onset diabetes has been made is how enthusiastically to treat the condition. Drugs should be kept as simple as possible because difficulties can arise from the patient's inability to adhere to complicated tablet regimes and the necessity for regular urine testing. Many old people, for economic reasons, live on a high-carbohydrate diet and there are sometimes problems of adjustment. Many 75-year-old diabetics are generally fit and well able to manage their own treatment. Sometimes, however, it is necessary to gain the help of some responsible relative or friend to supervise treatment. A general discussion will be necessary to explain the nature of the problem and possible dangers, including the side effects of drugs and complications of the disease.

Many cases of late-onset diabetes can be controlled by dietary measures. The diet should be simple, even if not quite correct, so that the patient can keep to it. It is easy to lose heart coping with a detailed and complicated regime. The diet should be in the region of 100–200 g of carbohydrate daily, a good starting point for most elderly patients being about 140 g of carbohydrate. The need to specify the amount of carbohydrate, however, is not really essential and nearly all elderly diabetics need only a no-sugar or ordinary reducing diet. The modern tendency is to restrict fats and cholesterol a little because diabetes is associated with a raised serum cholesterol and diabetics have enough trouble with their arteries without encouraging atheroma. A very strict low-cholesterol diet is probably unnecessary but perhaps the patient should know which foods contain most cholesterol so that they avoid eating more than a reasonable 'small normal' amount of such things as eggs and cream. Dieticians are usually very helpful in advising about these problems.

Many of the patients are also obese and the total calorie intake should be restricted. Obesity can contribute to the arterial complications of diabetes.

Hypoglycaemic agents are now an established part of the treatment of diabetes in old age. They are useful in controlling the glycaemic symptoms of the condition but there is some doubt whether they reduce the incidence of such complications as vascular disease. Two questions need answering about the use of these agents. First, in what type of patient should they be given and second, which preparation is best in old age? The type of case in which they are used usually is where diet alone does not control the diabetic symptoms. There are now a large number of hypoglycaemic agents available. They are of two types, the sulphonylureas (of which the most frequently used are probably chlorpropamide and tolbutamide) and the biguanides (metformin and phenformin). The most usual drug prescribed in old age is possibly chlorpropamide but there are some advantages in using tolbutamide in the first instance. It produces fewer gastrointestinal side effects and is shorter-acting, therefore reducing the likelihood of confusion induced by hypoglycaemia. The biguanides, particularly phenformin, should not be used for the aged as it is now recognized that they can predispose to lactic-acid acidosis.

All hypoglycaemic agents can cause side effects and these include gastrointestinal upset, allergic skin reactions and, more seriously, blood dyscrasias such as leukopenia and thrombocytopenia. Hypoglycaemic agents also react with other drugs being taken. With chlorpropamide and possibly other sulphonylureas, alcohol may interact and patients may experience hot flushes, giddiness, sickness and chest pain, 10–15 minutes after taking an alcoholic drink. It is necessary to warn patients about this possibility. Prolonged and unresponsive hypoglycaemia can occur with chlorpropamide in elderly patients. Beta blockers make recognition of hypoglycaemia more difficult, so if taken with hypoglycaemic tablets or insulin, attacks of hypoglycaemia become much more troublesome. There may be an increased incidence of hypothyroidism in patients taking long-term sulphonylurea treatment. Patients with hepatic and renal failure should, in theory, not be given oral hypoglycaemic agents. Congestive heart failure is a special problem and the question is sometimes raised as to whether oral hypoglycaemic agents should be used with thiazide diuretics. In practice, if the patient is in a stable situation it is probably safe, providing (1) special caution is taken when starting treatment or changing the dose; and (2) there is a constant awareness of the possibility that changes in the degree of failure, or reduction in hepatic or renal sufficiency, may change the diabetic state.

It is possible that a relatively low proportion of elderly patients require insulin treatment. There are new products now available and most elderly diabetics requiring insulin use these new highly purified insulins. Injections for old people need supervision and it is probably inadvisable for them to inject themselves. This must, however, depend upon individual circumstances and the availability of community nurses. A careful change of site is necessary to avoid necrotic ulcers forming. If insulin is required in a newly established case, stabilization is necessary in hospital because of the risks of hypoglycaemia. The danger of insulin therapy in an old person is the development of severe hypoglycaemia when meals are missed and incorrect doses are given. Clear instructions are absolutely essential. It is important to make sure that renal function is adequate.

Although late-onset diabetes may be considered to be a relatively mild condition, the complications are nevertheless common and serious. Therefore, in elderly people, these need especial attention whatever the type of diabetes. Ophthalmic, renal, vascular and neurological complications should be carefully monitored. Treatment is along the usual lines described in textbooks of medicine. At the earliest signs of difficulty, expert help should be sought and hypoglycaemic attacks should be treated in hospital. Chronic hypoglycaemia can easily be overlooked in elderly people since the only obvious symptoms are mild confusion, shivering or sweating. These occur frequently in old age from other causes.

There is now a shift in the care of elderly diabetic patients to the community. This has involved the creation of separate diabetic clinics in health centres where general practitioners can look after their own elderly diabetic patients. There are also some health visitors who have special training in diabetes and liaison nurses who maintain contact with the hospital diabetic clinics. Practice nurses are now being trained specifically to monitor elderly diabetic patients within practices. Regular follow-up is necessary to check the control of diabetes and to detect complications early. Foot problems should be avoided by regular visits to a chiropodist.

There is also the problem of elderly diabetics who hold driving licences. The risks of hypoglycaemia are such that it is very important that advice should be given about eating before driving for any distance and stopping frequently for snacks to step up the blood-sugar level. If the patient finds that he/she does not have any warning of hypoglycaemia, it is probably best to advise avoiding driving altogether.

Usually a long-established diabetic will not require any alteration in treatment with advancing age, but again it is important that the patient's condition is monitored. Each practice should have a check list of actions that should be undertaken at a follow-up clinic. This would include a review of the drugs, including possible side-effects, a check of blood sugar and glycosylated haemoglobin, a check of blood urea, a test for albumen in the urine, and checks on fundi, feet, reflexes and weight. The identification of diabetic retinopathy is becoming increasingly important because of the successful treatment of this condition by ophthalmic surgeons using laser therapy. It is also important at diabetic clinics to interview relatives and carers if possible so that any problems can be fully discussed and general support given.

COMMON CONDITIONS THAT IMPAIR MENTAL FUNCTION

Dementia

This is a condition that eventually results in a complete disruption of the personality. In the early stages there are minor degrees of intellectual difficulty with forgetfulness a prominent feature. There is a gradual reduction in the ability to learn new skills and adapt to changing environments. The emotions may be disorganized with inappropriate outbursts of crying or laughing. There is memory loss for recent events but happenings that occurred many years previously may be remembered with what appears to be astonishing accuracy. Objective tests show that these also are impaired, but not so much as new learning and therefore old learning appears relatively intact. There are two main types of dementia. First, Alzheimer's disease, which affects women more often than men and is characterized by a slowly progressive deterioration of personality and memory. Second, multi-infarct dementia, which is more common in men and follows a more stepwise deterioration of mental function. Each new cerebral infarct, often exhibiting physical signs, is followed by further reduction in cerebral function. There are several other rare dementing syndromes that, although theoretically important, are not practically significant. The management is difficult and along mainly supportive lines. Occasionally some mild sedation is helpful. Eventually the patient may have to be admitted to long-term care in hospital. The carers need a considerable amount of support in these circumstances. At present there is no effective drug therapy. The dementias are probably the biggest challenge to preventive health in old age. Despite the optimism generated by the aluminium story, there is little scope for primary or secondary prevention in Alzheimer's disease. There may, however, be developments in the genetic field that prove to be useful. Tertiary prevention can maintain maximum function where mental deterioration is present. Often the patient's physical condition is good. High blood pressure is a risk factor in both stroke and multi-infarct dementia. It is difficult to know whether lowering blood pressure in later rather than early life is preventive. In established cases of dementia, forward planning is clearly important and much can be done to manage patients at home but this often produces very considerable demands on relatives and carers.

Pseudo-dementia

This is a condition that resembles dementia but the underlying pathology is probably one of depression. It is characterized by guilt, self-reproach, paranoid and hypochondriacal behaviour. Apathy is present and also lack of concentration and impaired memory. However, the patient can briefly function at a higher, near-normal mental level, especially when under observation. Recognition of pseudo-dementia is important because of different treatment possibilities. Dementia is more likely if memory and cognitive impairment is reported before the depression. When tested, dementia patients tend to try to respond but give wrong answers, whereas depressed patients fail to try and say 'I don't know'. Dementia and depression can be present at the same time. This conjunction can be due to chance as both conditions are common, but multiple-infarcts in themselves can lead to both. The onset of dementia may be sensed by the patient and this can lead to reactive depression with ensuing self-neglect and social isolation. Depression can also lead to social neglect and resultant malnutrition causing vitamin deficiency, which may lead to confusion.

Acute confusion

The sudden onset of confusion in an elderly person is not an uncommon occurrence and ranks as an emergency that needs considerable skill and patience to manage effectively. The term 'acute confusional state' or 'delirium' is usually given to these episodes. Confusion is a clinical syndrome and not a diagnosis. Dementia can predispose an individual to confusion, but there are many other possibilities and it is always necessary to search for an underlying cause and remember that there may be several of these present at once. The list is lengthy and a full account can be found in a textbook of geriatric medicine. A summary of the causes is, however, given in Table 19.1.

Some acute crisis situations can also occur when there is a rapid deterioration of subacute or chronic confusion. They produce a very practical problem for community health and social workers. There are also background causes that contribute to the development of the crisis, but are not the illness itself. These are usually concerned with the provision of basic care to the patient and occur when this care is unavailable or withdrawn. Inadequacy of the services may also precipitate an acute situation and this has sometimes been called the 'GP frustration crisis'. The doctor dealing with the situation finds him/herself getting little help from either the hospital or social services, but is faced with continual representations from relatives, neighbours, shopkeepers and even town councillors to 'do something about' the old person. A great deal of strain results and the doctor is tempted to manipulate a crisis so that help can be obtained in a dramatic but perhaps not absolutely necessary form; this usually means an attempt to seek hospital admission. Sometimes this is, in effect, treatment for the doctor's problem! An example of this was the case of an old lady who regularly rang late each evening confessing some serious crime that she had committed earlier that day. She usually contacted the police as well, but was hurriedly told to get in touch with her doctor! In this type of category comes also what Tom Arie (1973) calls the 'preventive crisis', which may also be referred to as the 'Friday afternoon crisis'. Here, a

Table 19.1 Causes of acute confusional state

Intracranial	space-occupying lesion
	low-pressure encephalitis
	infection
	vascular episode
	trauma
Toxic	systemic infection
	gangrene
	alcohol
Endocrine	thyroid disease
	diabetes mellitus
Organ failure	renal
	hepatic
	respiratory
	anaemia
Vitamin deficiency	B group
Medication	altered response in old age
	withdrawal symptoms
	polypharmacy
Mental	presence of Alzheimer's Disease or multi-infarct dementia, especially when associated with chronic constipation, pain and discomfort
	depression
Social stress	acute worries regarding family ⎫
	harassment ⎬ especially when
	unfamiliar surroundings ⎪ dementia is present
	change in residence ⎭

Source: Williams (1988)

doctor sees a potentially difficult problem late on a Friday afternoon and being anxious to have it resolved, seeks urgent hospital admission. This may be a form of prevention and perhaps hospitals should recognize this; but equally, the doctor should be quite willing to accept the patient back into his care once the initial problem has been sorted out.

Acute confusional states usually have a rapid onset and often occur at night or in the early morning. Consciousness is clouded and disorientation is a marked feature. The mood is usually one of fear and anxiety, but occasionally the patient can be incongruously jocular, oblivious to reality. Speech is often incoherent and agitation with motor restlessness prominent. An important feature is the fluctuation of mental state over time. The acute confusion is often an episode in a more chronic situation in which the situations are suddenly exacerbated. In old people the state of sub-acute confusion is common. The episodes of acute confusion are usually short-lived with eventual recovery. This can depend on the underlying factor. Death may, however, be a possible outcome.

It is of prime importance to make a diagnosis of the patient's condition.

A very careful history needs to be taken and here a GP is in a privileged position. Knowledge of the background of previous illnesses, treatment currently being taken and the possibility of family stress is invaluable. The time course of the condition also needs to be known. Unfortunately, sometimes the GP is unaware of these because the condition has been unreported. The overall health of the patient needs assessing including noting physical illness and making an appreciation of the social and environmental circumstances. A very careful look needs to be taken for underlying background and precipitating causes. For instance, a special search must be made for respiratory and urinary-tract infection.

There is available in some districts a hospital service known as 'crisis-intervention'. Rather on the lines of an obstetric flying squad, a consultant psychiatrist, health visitor and community psychiatric nurse are prepared to turn out at any time, day or night, as well as at weekends to give help with an acute psychogeriatric crisis. Co-operation and assistance from the social services department are usually forthcoming. Expert help on the spot can be very useful for the GP and often it makes it possible to manage the situation at home by defusing a difficult situation and providing emergency care just at the right time.

Management of acute confusional state depends upon the underlying cause. In many instances hospital admission is necessary for investigation and treatment. When the episode is clearly associated with dementia, however, management at home has advantages because a move to a hospital environment can deepen the confusion. Often the patient is known to be suffering from the condition and, if not, a careful history from relatives or neighbours will usually indicate previous significant mental changes. A full history and examination is still necessary because other underlying illnesses may be present and be the principal cause of the confusion. In general practice few investigations are possible in the home, but testing the urine for sugar and infection are helpful; together with a blood test for cell count, haemoglobin, sugar, erythrocyte sedimentation rate, urea and electrolytes. Estimation of serum calcium level may be important because it is realized that primary hyperparathyroidism presents with acute confusion in elderly women. It is necessary to remember that calcium is raised in osteoporosis, neoplasma, Paget's Disease and thyrotoxicosis. Therefore a serum phosphate chloride and a haematocrit are also necessary.

If it is decided to manage the patient at home, it is probably useful to seek the help of a psychogeriatrician. The advantages are that it allows confirmation of the diagnosis and makes sure that there are no underlying causes present or further investigations necessary. It also provides the opportunity for a realistic plan of management to be formulated and secures at an early stage a link with the hospital so that there is knowledge of the patient's previous condition if eventual admission becomes necessary. Ideally, the consultation should take the form of a case conference at the patient's home where, as well as the specialist, the nursing and social worker members of the team should be present.

At that case conference, apart from physical examination and history, the following assessment must be made to determine the needs of the patient and the resources that are available to satisfy them. A nursing assessment will include note of other conditions that are present such as infections and ulcers, problems that may occur with diet, medication and dealing with a bedfast situation. A social assessment should include noting any difficulties that will occur in feeding, dressing, toileting, bathing the patient and with food preparation, laundry and cleaning of the house. Ensuring adequate heating will also be necessary. A suitable room for nursing the patient will be required and when assessing this the needs of other people, especially children, in the household should be considered. Safety is important and account must be taken of the risks of fires, electricity and gas, and the opportunities available for the patient to wander. The carers will need very careful support and it is necessary to assess how much help they can realistically give in providing twenty-four-hour cover. Financial assistance such as attendance allowance should be considered. Often voluntary services, for example Age Concern, and self-help groups such as the Alzheimer's Disease Society are useful.

In acute confusional state drugs should be used sparingly as they can make the situation worse. In a restless patient sedation may be used but the doses should be small and a careful watch kept for reactions. There are several possibilities, but most general practitioners tend to use the one they know best. The three most useful are haloperidol, thioridazine and chlormethiazole. Haloperidol is effective and has the advantage of decreased risks of hypotension. It should only be used for a short time because it may produce extrapyramidal side effects. Anti-Parkinsonian drugs should be avoided because of the risk of causing increased confusion. Thioridazine is also useful; it has a low instance of Parkinsonian side-effects but can give rise to postural hypotension. Chlormethiazole is also used in patients with confusional agitation and is relatively free of side effects in a low dose. For all these drugs it is essential in the young old to start with about half the dose of the normal adult and in the old old and those of low weight with a quarter of the normal dose. Careful monitoring of the effects is essential, especially excess drowsiness, which can lead to falls and incontinence. In some circumstances if there has been any hint of poor nutrition, vitamin supplements may be helpful.

Particular problems arise where the patient lives alone and sometimes hospital admission is necessary just for this reason. But occasionally when the mental problem is severe or the patient refuses to co-operate, serious difficulties of care result. Use of provisions under the Mental Health Act are sometimes necessary in these circumstances.

Finally, long-term supervision is usually necessary once the initial crisis period is passed. Established nursing and social-worker services need to be reassessed and placed on a maintenance basis. Short-term respite may be needed for carers. Although not common in the UK, boarding out of mentally sick old people in foster homes is used in some countries to provide such care. Some private homes are now caring for mentally confused old patients. Existing home accommodation may be inappropriate and occasionally it is best to rehouse the patient or make adaptations to the existing building. If this is impossible and the person lives alone, permanent admission to a welfare home, particularly one specializing in the care of people with a mental disorder, may be the only possibility.

An open mind needs to be kept on all the options and it might be that at some future date, hospital admission may be necessary because of a rapidly changing clinical condition, or failure to respond to treatment. Day-hospital care may sometimes be helpful and has the advantage of avoiding the difficulties associated with admission. Relief for relatives is often considerable when this can be arranged and there is the added advantage of others being able to watch the patient's response to treatment more closely.

Finally, the preventive aspects of the community-care team's work are important when considering confusional problems in elderly people. The aim should be to recognize intellectual impairment at an early stage. This can be done by having an alert attitude to old people presenting at the surgery. The importance of knowing what to look for at an early stage in the development of mental illness cannot be overstressed. Failure of recent memory, changing behaviour, alteration in emotional response and depression are features that should be noted.

There are also certain at-risk groups that are more likely to develop mental illness in its widest sense and they need special surveillance. They include people living alone, the recently bereaved and those with social problems, particularly of finance and housing. Patients recently discharged from hospital or welfare homes may well find difficulty in adapting to life in the community and sometimes relapse, developing mental symptoms. The family doctor is in a special position to be able to recognize the early deterioration of a person's mental condition because of his/her knowledge of the previous personality. Despite this it is possible that crises will occur, but with preventive action their frequency should be reduced.

Affective disorders

These are common in old age and account for up to half the admissions to mental hospitals in the over-65 age group. They consist of the manic-depressive illnesses and are associated with a dysfunction in the patient's emotional state. Deterioration of intellect may, of course, also be present. The individual presents with a weary air of overall depression and there is often an associated degree of apathy. Patients may be fearful for the health of themselves and their relatives and show hypochondriacal symptoms. They may worry even more about their own financial and housing difficulties. There may be physical components to the illness, including complaints of lack of sleep, poor appetite and headache. A small percentage, perhaps between 5 and 10% of these patients, exhibit the manic phase of the illness. These people are hyperexcitable, often agitated and highly talkative, going to great lengths to describe the importance of their achievements. Outrageous activities may be embarked upon such as spending a large quantity of money on items such as a new car or a quite unnecessary pieces of furniture.

Suicide is a real danger in a depressed old person, the incidence being higher than in younger age groups. They feel a sense of unworthiness and no longer want to live: they talk about 'doing away with themselves' and this is particularly likely to happen when they have recently lost a spouse or other relative. They often say they would be better off if they could join the lost loved one. Occasionally a depressed old person is able to camouflage the depression quite successfully by confining conversations to the past and being unwilling to talk about the problems of the present. By so doing, the feelings of sadness that are constantly present are blocked out by more pleasant memories of past life.

Paraphrenia

Sometimes patients present in old age with symptoms that are predominantly paranoid, most often a feeling of being watched or persecuted in some way. Professor Anderson (1971) describes the patient as 'classically a woman, often unmarried, and frequently affected by disorders of either vision or hearing'. Indeed, deafness is said to be very potent in producing these symptoms. The patients, who might have had paranoid traits throughout life, develop delusions in old age, particularly about neighbours, whom they see as a threat. Others develop fantasy ideas about sex and imagine that they are being watched whilst undressing or even have worries about being molested.

Acute-anxiety state

This is also common in old age. The patients present with the usual worried and agitated demeanour. Bodily symptoms are common and the patient often complains of sweating, faintness, rapid pulse rate and headache. Indeed, physical symptoms may predominate. There are usually predisposing causes such as financial and housing worries. Harassment may be a problem and old people, particularly those living alone, may be easily upset by the uncalled-for activity of certain neighbours. Particularly unpleasant cases occur when old women are attacked and even raped either in their own home or outside. Fear of this type of assault can easily induce an acute-anxiety state.

Behaviour disorders and personality changes

It has been said that personality defects that are present in earlier life are exaggerated as one grows older and this can be seen quite commonly in the community. A person who has been a little on the ungenerous side can become, with age, positively mean and miserly. Similarly, one who has been occasionally short-tempered can become extremely awkward and unpleasant in old age. A person who was constantly quarrelling with neighbours can take this to extremes as the years advance. Enemies created in earlier life can take on a more important and sinister aspect. This may apply to relatives. Sometimes there have been hidden jealousies between members of the same family and these come to the surface in old age. These personality changes lead to the patient becoming more inward-looking; the circle of friendships diminishes, and in the end the old person lives a hermit's life and can be quite unapproachable and difficult to help.

There is described amongst hospital in-patients a condition of institutional neurosis in which they show apathy and loss of initiative. This is said to be one reason for keeping people out of hospital. It can, however, also happen at home and the neurosis can equally well occur when patients are 'institutionalized' in the confines of their own houses.

Although old people very rarely consult with sexual problems, the family may come to the doctor with stories of aberrant sexual behaviour. An elderly man may suddenly develop a preoccupation with sex and this may produce difficulties with female relatives or helpers. Sometimes indecent exposure is a problem and occasionally overt sexual advances may be made to any member of the opposite sex who happens to be present. Occasionally, these take the form of indecent assault on children. A sexual problem may also manifest itself in quite unrealistic jealousies and can result in physical violence.

Alcoholism is occasionally seen for the first time in old age and there may be associated features of anxiety or depression. It is necessary when dealing with an acute episode of confusion to bear in mind the possibility of this problem and look for the tell-tale evidence of large numbers of bottles scattered around the house or in the dustbins.

Obsessive neurosis may also develop in old people and they can become completely dominated by such things as cleanliness and the position of various pieces of furniture around the house. The timing of meals will have to be exact, as perhaps will the amount of sleep taken. Sometimes, such obsessions concern physical health and the patient may become absolutely fixed on the idea that he/she has got a cancer and frequent visits are paid to the doctor with a whole variety of symptoms. Many X-rays and consultant opinions are called for and the patient, within a few months, can pass rapidly from one hospital department to another. Very little seems to be able to convince these people that they are, in fact, physically well.

THE LAW AND VULNERABLE ELDERLY PEOPLE

Incapacity in old age brings with it the need on occasion for both protection and representation. The law is inevitably concerned with these issues and the subject is of some complexity. The Age Concern book, *The Law and Vulnerable Elderly People* (Greengross, 1986), gives an excellent account of the law as it stands and discusses some of the issues. The law has recently changed regarding the power of attorney, which has improved the practical management of these situations.

A power of attorney is the arrangement whereby a person gives authority to another or others to act on his/her behalf. It is used, for instance, when the infirmity is physical and an elderly person has difficulty in writing a cheque. Since the *Enduring Powers of Attorney Act* (1985) came into force on 10 March 1986 there are now two forms of power: the power of attorney and the enduring power of attorney. The power of attorney enables some other person to sign documents in the name of the person who has been given the power. Authority given to the donee is wide, but it can be limited to a particular purpose. Once the power has been executed, it can be produced to interested persons and the signature of the donee will then be accepted in place of that of the donor. The power of attorney should, however, only be used when the donor is of full mental capacity and if the old person's mental state deteriorates, the existing power will become invalid. This caused problems in the past and because of this the *Enduring Powers of Attorney Act* came into force. It followed the Law Commission's report *The Incapacitated Principle*, which recommended that the law be changed so that certain powers of attorney could continue after the donor becomes mentally incapacitated. Enduring power of attorney is designed to ensure that the nature of the power is understood by donor and the attorney. It has been of considerable benefit both to the legal profession and to anyone else dealing with elderly persons. To deal with the problem of mental incapacity, the *Enduring Powers of Attorney Act* provides that a power of attorney executed under the provisions of that act does not expire when the donor of the power becomes mentally incapable, but continues during the incapacity.

The enduring power of attorney is a fairly simple form. The attorney appointed can be either an individual or two persons jointly and they can be given full authority to act or their authority can be limited to certain things. It would be normal in most cases where the attorney is a close relative and probably an ultimate beneficiary of the estate, for the person to be given general authority to deal with all the donor of the power's property and affairs. Specific restrictions can, however, be inserted into the power but – and this is the crucial difference from the old powers – the power states that 'I intend that this Power should continue even if I become mentally incapable.' The donor is required to state that he/she has read the notes in Part A of the form that set out full details of what the attorney can do, and in particular set out that the power will continue if the donor becomes mentally incapable. The document is simply signed by the donor in the presence of a witness and the attorney is required to sign also to say that they realize that when the donor has become mentally incapable they are under a duty to apply to the court for the registration of the power of attorney under the *Enduring Powers of Attorney Act*. As, and when, the donor of the power becomes, or is thought to be becoming, mentally incapable, the power is registered with the Court of Protection. Since the attorney appointed is chosen by the elderly person themselves there is not the difficulty and formality that used to be experienced with the appointment of a receiver by the Court of Protection. The power can, of course, be cancelled by the donor at any time before it has been registered.

If elderly people cannot manage their own affairs because of mental disorder, and where an enduring power of attorney is not in existence, it is necessary to go to the Court of Protection, which exists to safeguard the elderly person's interests. The Court has existed in one form or another for six hundred years, but it is now regulated by the *Mental Health Act* (1983) and the *Court of Protection Rules* (1984). In June 1985 there were 22 545 people under the Court of Protection. It is estimated that 75% were over 60, many living in residential homes or in Part III accommodation, others in hospital or nursing home and some in their own or relatives' homes.

The Court's responsibility is for financial matters. The office is in Store Street, London, WC1E 7BP and a letter to the Chief Clerk will produce guidance for relatives of those in this situation. In effect, once the case has been properly investigated and the incapacity of the elderly person established by written evidence from the appropriate medical practitioner, all the affairs of the elderly person are placed under the supervision of the Court of Protection and property cannot be disposed of, nor can income or assets be dealt with, unless the Court of Protection agrees. The Court will usually appoint some person known as a receiver, who is often a close relative or in default a friend or professional adviser, to deal, under its instruction, with the elderly person's property. All transactions in the financial affairs of the person concerned must be dealt with in this way. To avoid frequent applications to the Court, normally an order is made for weekly payments for the benefit of the elderly person, but any disposal of assets such as a house or investments will need the specific sanction of the Court of Protection. The legal costs of obtaining such an order and of administering it are normally dealt with out of the estate of the person concerned.

MOBILITY

Assessment of mobility is a very important aspect of the examination of an old person. Loss of mobility can be partial or complete. The prevalence of totally bedfast old people is not high, but increases with advancing age. Relative immobility, which often means that the person is housefast, is a common cause of reduced effective health. Functional ability is all important and before examination of the limbs and joints, it is necessary to find out what the old person can actually do. Can the patient do the following things: walk unaided or only with a frame, tripod or support from furniture; get out of bed or a chair; stoop to pick things up from the floor; undertake basic personal tasks? It is also helpful to know whether the patient can use public transport, shop and enjoy hobbies and social contact.

If diminished mobility has been established by functional assessment, possible causes should be sought by examination. Pain, stiffness and swelling of the joints, and weakness, wasting, tremor or rigidity of the limbs, if present, are obvious, and a patient's stance may also be awkward and unsteady. Movements may lack co-ordination. A weak grip may interfere with efficient use of walking aids. Examination of the feet sometimes reveals gnarled toenails and twisted joints that hinder walking. Improperly fitting shoes sometimes also contribute to immobility.

Immobility is always a feature of a disorder. By itself it does not constitute a diagnosis. Pain and weakness are the main reasons for the difficulty in movement, with perhaps mental apathy contributing to the overall inertia. Pain, which must never be accepted as normal in old age, may arise from bones, muscles or joints. Bone causes include osteoporosis, osteomalacia, Paget's disease and malignancies. Skeletal causes include osteoarthitis, rheumatoid arthritis and, less frequently, gout. Many minor muscular reasons, such as fibrositis, can cause pain and immobility. An illness that affects elderly people particularly is polymyalgia rheumatica. This is more common in women and associated with pain and stiffness in the neck, spreading to the shoulder muscles and also occasionally the gluteal and thigh muscles. The patient may also have generalized symptoms such as headaches, sweating and anorexia. The condition is sometimes associated with temporal arteritis and in both, the erythrocyte sedimentation rate is raised. The illness lasts for a few months and is likely to be recurrent. The treatment is by using steroids, often in large doses. The dose is then reduced according to the level of ESR and the relief of symptoms.

The condition of the feet of old people is important as disorders easily impede mobility. Bunions associated with hallux valgus may be extremely painful, as are corns and callouses. Toenail deformity may make walking extremely difficult. Recently the prevalence of fungal infection of the feet of patients in geriatric wards has been highlighted and in a sample of patients almost all had positive cultures of certain fungal organisms.

Neurological disease can produce actual muscle wasting and lack of co-ordination. Two examples of this are motor neurone disease and Parkinson's disease. The latter condition is characterized by lack of movement, rigidity and tremor. The face shows a masklike appearance and dementia may be an associated condition. A shuffling gait, consisting of a few small steps and a tendency to lean forward, with difficulty in stopping, is frequently seen. Generalized clumsiness is often present with difficulty in dressing and undressing a marked feature. The rigidity may be severe and the cogwheel effect of a series of small jerks when moving the elbow may be demonstrated. The tremor starts in the hand and is coarse, becoming increased when a voluntary movement is undertaken, but disappears during sleep. Motor neurone disease is characterized by wasting of the muscles of all four limbs. Fasciculation or fine movements in the muscles can be seen and the reflexes are brisk. The weakness associated with the muscle wasting can sometimes become severe and can lead to considerable difficulty. This can be particularly burdensome when the mental state remains unimpaired and patients who have previously been able to look after themselves, and even drive a car, find it extremely frustrating to be limited by muscular weakness. The tongue and throat muscles can be affected, giving rise to difficulties with salivation, swallowing and nutrition.

Disorders of the heart and lung can contribute to immobility by causing breathlessness, ankle swelling, chest pain or pain in the legs on walking. General debility may result from endocrine, renal and blood diseases, and reduce a patient's ability to move around. A patient's mental state, if impaired, can also contribute to inertia, and visual and hearing difficulties can have the same effect. Oversedation and the side effects of some drugs not infrequently limit mobility. Occasionally old people can suddenly go 'off their feet' and for no obvious reason become bedfast. These cases are analagous to the 'failure to thrive' syndrome in infants, and the cause may be equally difficult to find. Sometimes diseases such as a chest infection are responsible. More than one pathology may contribute to immobility, and such conditions as obesity and anaemia often exacerbate the problem. Extreme old age itself can influence movements (disuse atrophy) although it is often surprising how spry many 90-year olds can be.

It can be seen that there are many causes of immobility. There must be motivation to move out of the house or at least out of the chair. Sometimes an inconveniently placed house can psychologically deter an old person from making the effort to venture outside. Management has to take all these aspects into account. However, it is important that full medical examination is carried out in order to detect underlying conditions. Physical illnesses must be treated, if they exist. Chiropody may be all that is necessary in some circumstances, but occasionally, full rehabilitation services may be needed to mobilize the patient. Provision of aids, appliances and modifications to the house are often helpful, particularly as part of a general programme of physiotherapy. Stimulating an old person mentally by encouraging interest in an outside activity or hobby can change a housefast isolate into a more active member of the community. Transfer to ground-floor accommodation near a shopping precinct may enable an old person once more to undertake independent shopping. In all this, the role of the community physiotherapist is very important. Help from him/her can be obtained during the initial assessment and also when planning management. Physiotherapy in the home plays a crucial part in returning an old person to full mobility or achieving the best possible result. The effect that a good physiotherapist can have on the morale and confidence of an old person is impressive to see.

FALLS

Falls are a major hazard of old age and a common cause of injury and sometimes death. Clarke (1972), when studying falls, found that nearly three-quarters of them occurred in or near the patient's home and about one-fifth further afield. These latter take place almost exclusively near roads, particularly on pavements, kerbs and pedestrian crossings, where distraction by traffic or uneven surfaces are commonly causal factors. Getting on and off buses can also be a hazard. The remainder of falls take place usually in welfare homes or hospital and it is less common for them to occur in such places as churches, shops and places of work.

Causes of falls

Clarke (1972) describes three main types of fall mechanism:

1. Accidental falls: here the event is determined by environmental factors only, for example, slipping on an icy surface or tripping over a rug or a mat.
2. Symptomatic falls: here the cause is due to factors within the patient

and can result from either fits or faints. In this group are also falls caused by dizziness or light-headedness.
3. Mixed-type falls: here both environmental and patient factors are combined.

Of the accidental variety there are many possible causes; they include trips, slips and being knocked over by a vehicle or another person. Symptomatic falls can be caused, as stated above, by fits or faints. Grand mal-type epileptic fits might be due to pre-existing idiopathic epilepsy or to cerebrovascular disease, intracranial tumour, trauma or hypoglycaemia. Fainting attacks without the characteristics of a fit may be due to transient ischaemic attack, cardiac infarction, a Stokes–Adams attack or postural hypotension. Another cause is the so-called 'drop attack' whose nature is still rather obscure. Characteristically, in these attacks, the patient, most commonly a woman, falls suddenly because without warning, the legs go weak and flaccid. There is no loss of consciousness but the unsteadiness of the legs often persists for some time. Falls also occur at night when the patient is wandering. These may be due to postural hypotension occurring when a person gets out of bed quickly, following a sudden urge to pass urine. A patient may be confused at night because of too heavy sedation, or restless because of too little sedation. Both circumstances can lead to nocturnal wanderings and cause falls. Overuse of alcohol by old people, a problem that is perhaps increasing, can also be contributory. Patients with general debility and frailness are more likely to fall, particularly if they also suffer from Parkinson's disease and especially when this is combined with poor vision. Falls are also more likely after a period in bed because of illness.

It seems that there is a physiological decline in postural control with advancing age and falls are often associated with impaired balance. Old people are unable to correct themselves once they have stumbled, and there is a higher proportion of falls from causes other than tripping in patients over 75 years old.

Management

Management of acute fall depends of course on the injuries sustained. Ideally, an eye-witness account of the episode should be obtained so that if there is a possibility that the fall was due to a fit investigation can be undertaken. This could be very extensive if all the causes of a fit in an old person were to be eliminated, and common sense is necessary when deciding what tests to undertake. Help from a consultant geriatrician is usually to be recommended. Again, when the cause of the fall has been a faint of some type, a search for disease causes should be made. Some of these conditions can be treated and it is important that this should be done if possible.

It is important to look at the patient's social circumstances. Safety in the home must be assessed and the arrangement of the patient's living area may need adjustment. Sometimes it is necessary where a person is having frequent falls and is living alone, to arrange transfer to welfare accommodation or to warden-supervised housing.

Prevention of falls

The aim should be, if possible, to prevent falls. Clarke (1972) lists simple ways of approaching the problem and these are summarized here.

1. Removal of hazards in the home. In many instances these are obvious, but particular attention should be paid to loose rugs, carpets with holes and uneven surfaces. A good standard of lighting is essential and high wattage bulbs should be used. Handrails may be fitted to aid the old person's movement. All fires should be protected by fireguards.
2. Preservation of good health and confidence. When a patient has had a fall, assessment is necessary so that treatable conditions can be remedied. Poor vision should be corrected. Careful rehabilitation after illness or injury should reduce the possibility of further accident.
3. Wearing of appropriate footwear. Rubber and crepe soles are unsatisfactory in wet and icy conditions. Non-slip or leather soles are preferable.
4. Special care outdoors. In winter, when conditions are bad, high-risk persons should remain indoors. If it is necessary to go out, they should be accompanied and routes should be chosen where there is likely to be the least danger from distraction by traffic. They should cross busy roads on pedestrian crossings if at all possible, and carry shopping in a wheeled container. Care should be taken when boarding and alighting from public transport. A careful watch should be kept for uneven surfaces and care taken at kerbs.
5. Awareness of the dangers of sudden changes in posture. Patients should be careful when getting in and out of bed or chairs and instructed to do this slowly.
6. Monitoring of night sedation. Careful attention is needed to the level of night sedation prescribed for an old person, since this may be more a cause of falls than a help. Indeed, all drug therapy for patients with falls should be reviewed. Night sedation should, however, be adequate so that nocturnal wanderings are avoided.

It is obviously essential to identify patients who are at risk of falling. Screening old people at clinics for elderly people can help and note can be made of patients with a history of falling. Preventive measures can then be instituted and the patients educated about the various safety precautions.

VISION FAILURE

Over the past twenty years there has been a change in the age prevalence of blindness. These days, most severely defective vision occurs amongst elderly people. Visual failure can be an important cause of loss of independence and result in social isolation. With increasing blindness, mobility becomes more difficult and an old person is deprived of hobbies such as gardening, watching television and visiting the cinema. Vision can be quickly and simply assessed by asking patients if they can read a newspaper, watch television or recognize the details of a photograph or picture.

Comparatively few people become blind suddenly and there is likely to be a gradual deterioration of vision over several years. This is always due to disease and old age alone is not a cause of blindness. The commonest diseases leading to failing vision are cataract, macular degeneration and chronic glaucoma. Sudden loss of vision, when it occurs, is usually due to acute glaucoma, occlusion of the central retinal artery or vein or a detached retina. Chronic open-angle glaucoma produces gradual loss of vision. Many of these conditions are treatable.

Cataracts, which may originate much earlier in life, develop slowly and are often symmetrical. Successful extraction and later optical correction using contact lenses is possible in old people, but the majority are more happily corrected with spectacles as contact lenses are only suitable for the dextrous and motivated; best of all from the optic point of view, and increasingly used, are acrylic lenticuli implanted into the eye when a cataract is removed.

Senile macular degeneration with pigmentation of the macula is difficult to treat, although, as the periphery is not affected, complete blindness does not occur. Many cases of macular degeneration are helped by low-vision aids, for example telescopic glasses or simple hand magnifiers.

Diabetic retinopathy can be halted to a certain extent by careful control of the disease. Partial ablation of the diabetic retina, either by light coagulation or laser therapy, is useful in many cases as it delays retinopathy by cutting down the oxygen needs, hence allowing the ailing vasculature to maintain the important central area.

Acute glaucoma is not very common and usually presents as an emergency. The angle is closed in these cases and the second eye is invariably at risk, hence the need for prophylactic peripheral iridectomy. Early symptoms include blurring of vision and the perception of 'halo' effects round lights. Glaucomatous haloes are specifically rainbow-lined, the so-called 'rainbow rings'. Monochromic haloes around lights are common and may indicate cataract. Vision is subsequently lost and symptoms vary from an ache to severe pain. The intraocular tension is increased and the pupil is usually fixed, oval and dilated, rather than distorted. The chronic, open-angle type that occurs in old people is more common and much more insidious in onset. The visual field is lost, often to a remarkable extent, before the situation is recognized. It is important that this loss should be appreciated as it may be highly dangerous to old people, for instance, when crossing roads. Apart from field loss and raised intra-ocular pressure, cupping of the optic disc is present. When examining old people, it is useful to check the ocular tension and to do a simple visual-field test. Sometimes the condition is genetically determined and relatives of patients with glaucoma should be examined. Treatment is specialized and surgery is recommended for acute glaucoma. Timoptol (MSD) 0.25% is the treatment of choice in chronic open-angle glaucoma.

Despite the efficiency of the drops and often because of poor com-pliance in elderly people, many patients with these conditions become permanently partially sighted or blind. Even in these cases, much can be done to help. The first essential is to place the patient's name on the Blind Register. A certificate of registration (BD8 in England and Wales and BP1 in Scotland) must first be completed by a consultant ophthalmologist and forwarded to the local social services department. A social worker then interviews the blind person to explain the voluntary nature of registration and the benefits available. For registration, it is necessary to define the degree of blindness or partial-sightedness. These special criteria are fully set out in Form BD8.

Registration in working adults has considerable effect on the help they get with jobs and training, but this is rarely applicable to elderly people. Social services departments are responsible for social care of elderly people on the Register. Casework is available, as is help with travel, supply of white canes and 'talking books'. Rehabilitation centres sometimes cater for newly blind old people. Some voluntary organizations are particularly interested in the blind and their assistance should be sought.

Despite this help, many old people with failing vision find it difficult to cope. There is a limit to what can be achieved by re-education and perhaps it is wiser to aim at only realistic objectives. First, the newly blind old person should be encouraged to walk around the house, making sure that no dangerous objects are in the way. The furniture should remain in the same place so that the old person can learn the way around and gain confidence. Dressing and undressing can be made easier by using clothes that have few buttons and making use of zip fasteners. Shoes should be slip-on rather than laced. Shaving should be undertaken by an electric razor and eating and drinking can be helped by special utensils. New interests can be encouraged such as radio, records and tape recordings. Talking books are helpful and, for the partially sighted, books with large print can be obtained from most libraries. Good lighting is essential.

It is perhaps too late for most old people to learn Braille but there are simpler types of tactile reading such as the Moon system that may be possible. There is much sympathy in society generally for the blind and an old person so affected should be encouraged to persist in social activities and remain a part of the community.

DEAFNESS

The prevalence of deafness increases with age. In a survey of over-75-year olds, 9% were effectively totally deaf and many more could hear only the shouted voice (Williams *et al.*, 1972). Often they were prepared to tolerate the disability without seeking help. Unlike blindness, deafness attracts little sympathy. This adds to the sufferer's problems and because of embarrassment, they may become socially isolated and even develop paranoid symptoms.

Very simple tests will assess an old person's hearing ability. The responses to a ticking watch, a whispered, normal and shouted voice, give an adequate estimate of hearing. The basic types of hearing loss are conductive deafness, nerve deafness and a combination of the two, mixed deafness. The Rinne test distinguishes conductive and nerve deafness. This is carried out by holding a vibrating 512 Hz tuning fork close to the ear canal and then immediately pressing the base of the fork on the bone behind. It is heard better by the bone in conductive losses. The opposite is the case in nerve deafness (and the normal ear). A false negative Rinne, in which a tuning fork placed on the mastoid process is heard better by air conduction occurs in severe sensory-neural losses and is attributed to sound being conducted across the skull to the opposite cochlea.

Wax may only muffle otherwise good hearing but can considerably aggravate poor hearing. Good benefit is obtained by syringing away wax, which, if hard, should be softened by a few days' use of olive oil. When syringing, it is necessary to be sure that the water is approximately body temperature. If too hot or cold it can cause troublesome temporary unsteadiness.

Hearing is dependent on sound vibrations being collected by the eardrums and transmitted by the three small bones (ossicles) of the middle ear to the cochlea, which contains the nerve endings of the hearing nerve. Conductive hearing loss is due to disorder of the drum or ossicles. Two common causes are a perforated drum or osscular adhesions, both legacies of infection. Conductive hearing loss may also be due to disease of the ear canal. Another cause is otosclerosis, an inherited tendency to new bone formation, which interferes with the stapes, the innermost ossicle. This, however, is uncommon in elderly people and usually presents earlier in life. Nerve deafness in elderly people is usually due to presbyacusis – a word meaning gradual degeneration of the cochlea. Noise-induced hearing loss from previous noisy work commonly adds to presbyacusis. Less common causes are trauma, other inherited disorders, Menière's disease and Paget's disease of the skull.

Noises in the ears and head (tinnitus) may accompany any type of deafness. In elderly people, while this cannot be cured it may be treated with appropriate advice and indeed a hearing aid may be an effective way of helping control tinnitus by providing more sound for the patient with the condition. Occasionally in elderly people, provision of a tinnitus masker may be of benefit. Explanation and reassurance concerning its benign nature may help patients to come to terms with the condition.

Very substantial help is given to most deaf people by hearing aids but normal hearing can never be restored. There are two types available: those worn behind the ear and body-worn aids that may be necessary when severe deafness is present. Both are available to elderly people on the National Health Service. Conductive deafness responds rather better than nerve deafness. It is essential to make sure that the old person knows how to use the device and a certain degree of teaching is necessary to bring maximum benefit. This is normally given at the hospital hearing-aid clinics. When talking to a deaf person it is important to speak clearly and it is preferable to face the listener. Many people, even though they have not been formally instructed in lip-reading skills, are able to utilize lip and facial information in what is being said.

REFERENCES

Anderson, W.F. (1971) *Practical Management for the Elderly.* Blackwell Scientific Publications, Oxford and Edinburgh.

Arie, T. (1973) Dementia in the elderly: diagnosis and assessment. *Br. Med. J.,* **4**, 540–3.

Clarke, A.N.G. (1972) Falls in old age. *Modern Geriatrics,* **2** (6), 332–6.

Greengross, S. (ed.) (1986) *The Law and Vulnerable Elderly People,* Age Concern, London.

Orme, M. (1988) Leading Article. Aspirin all round. *Br. Med. J.,* **296**, 307–8.

Thompson, M.K. (1986) The case for developmental gerontology – Thompson's Octad. *J. R. Coll. Gen. Pract.,* **39**, 29–32.

Williams, E.I. (1988) Crisis management of acute confusion. *Mims Magazine,* pp. 87–93, 1 March.

Williams, E.I., Bennett, F.M., Nixon, J.V. *et al.* (1972) Socio-medical survey of patients over 75 in general practice. *Br. Med. J.,* **2**, 445–8.

20 *Ethical issues in the community*

A greater understanding of the problems of caring for old people in the community has highlighted some ethical problems that may occur. Many of these centre around such issues as respect for the person, degrees of acceptable risk, confidentiality and matters of life and death. This section will examine these in relation particularly to the family doctor working in the community, but they may confront any health or social worker. Instead of analysing the problems individually, they will be discussed in relation to actual patients whose histories will be described and the ethical problems identified. Each of these cases is intended to demonstrate a particular problem, but as always in medicine there is a considerable amount of overlap and often two or three ethical dilemmas are confronted on the same situation. Nine cases will now be described and the under-lying ethical problems and common features will be discussed at the end of the chapter. The names have, of course, been changed.

1. The Lomax couple – 'through whose eyes are we looking?'

Mrs Lomax is aged 84 and her husband is six years her junior. They have been married for over 50 years. They had two sons, both of whom were married and both of whom have died within the past ten years. The only relative they have any contact with is a grandson who lives 10 miles away. The health of both is bad. Mrs Lomax has chronic heart failure, generalized osteoarthritis and an irritating skin rash. Her arthritis makes her immobile and she is only able to shuffle around the house using either a Zimmer frame or a walking stick. Mr Lomax is virtually blind, but otherwise reasonably healthy and mobile. He suffers from early senile dementia and is forgetful and occasionally confused. They live in a ground-floor flat in a block purposely built for elderly people. Unfortun-ately they have few contacts with their neighbours. They get help from social services in the form of meals on wheels and home help.

A central feature of their life is constant quarrelling. This seems to have been present for many years but is, in old age, particularly distressing to those around. They both, however, manage to deal with this and it may be an important part of their relationship. In effect, Mrs Lomax acts as the brain and the eyes and Mr Lomax as the hands and the mobility. The two are in a state of brittle equilibrium and just able to attend to their domestic and personal requirements.

Comment
This case presents a number of awkward dilemmas for the doctor. Neither of the patients is receiving adequate medical care. Treatment is unreliable as tablets are not taken regularly despite daily visits by the district nurse. This non-compliance is due to a combination of apathy, forgetfulness, poor vision and confusion. Outside observers would say that both patients should be in hospital or at least in welfare accommodation where treatment can be properly supervised. Nevertheless, they are just coping and the question arises as to what should be the aim of medical care: therapeutic perfection, or patient satisfaction with the present state? Outsiders would also say that the pair are unhappy. One only needs to listen to their constant complaints and incessant quarrelling. This, however, may be absolutely necessary to their wellbeing and in no way detracts from their state of happiness. Without this stimulus, life may lack its spice and hence not be worth living.

Even more difficult is the social aspect. The house is dirty, untidy and a minefield of hazards. Cooking facilities are basic and potentially dangerous. If it were not for meals on wheels, nutrition would be totally inadequate – again all very strong reasons to move the pair into some form of supervised care.

Yet through whose eyes do we observe their predicament? To the much younger eyes of the doctor, nurse and social worker the conditions under which the Lomax couple live are wholly unacceptable. How could anyone live in such chaos it might be asked? Especially as one of these is immobile and the other is blind. Yet to these people this is the accepted norm: the environment that is understood. They support each other after a fashion and they have survived. How much should one meddle with such a situation? Would interference really be in the best interests of these two old people, or would a move be purely to satisfy the anxieties of the professional carers who experience a sense of unease when observing what might be described as neglect? Is it reasonable, ethically, to carry such a burden of responsibility, realizing that the best is not being achieved for these patients? Who judges what is best? How far is collusion allowable? The apathy of old age, along with the blunted understanding of early dementia, denies reality. Doctors have inbuilt into their value systems a duty to respect the person they are treating; to share with the patients a knowledge of the problems, the possibilities, the decisions and their implications. But who is the person the doctor must respect? Is it the person the doctor knew ten or twenty years ago, articulate and well-integrated, or is it the person he/she now sees?

In the case of the Lomax couple the problem can become compounded when one develops an illness that makes him/her unable to fulfil their part of the partnership arrangement. If, for instance, Mrs Lomax goes into heart failure and needs bed rest, it means that she becomes unable to supervise Mr Lomax in the tasks of general housework. Does the doctor admit her to hospital and leave him to manage alone, or admit him to a welfare home where he would be unhappy? Alternatively, can he treat her at home and risk disaster?

What are the priorities in this situation? Is it the equilibrium that they have and that would be broken if either of them were taken away from their home for any length of time, or is it the health of Mrs Lomax? Would Mr Lomax in fact survive if he were admitted to a welfare home? Unfortunately, the answers to these questions are not predictable at the time when decisions have to be made. Whatever happens, it is likely that decisions taken in favour of one will not benefit the other. Doctors are, however, expected to make these decisions. The general principle has always been to preserve life, but the dilemma sometimes arises, and it does so particularly in this case, as to whose life it is best to preserve.

2. Tom Barlow – 'defeat'

Tom Barlow is a widower aged 88. He lives alone in a state of some personal neglect. His condition is dirty and that of his house squalid. He lives in a downstairs room where he sleeps, eats and attends to his toilet. There are no visible carers, but it is probable that there are relatives in the district who refuse to have anything to do with him because of his condition. The only contact Mr Barlow has with the outside world is through a neighbour who visits on a very irregular basis. His main diet is baked beans. He will not have home-help or meals-on-wheels services, although both have been offered by social workers on several occasions. In fact, he is averse to any type of external assistance and certainly does not want to move from his house. He is ill with chronic bronchitis and heart failure. He has been offered treatment for this by the doctor and has also been offered hospital admission. He refuses to take tablets except on a very irregular basis. His compliance with any type of therapeutic plan is almost non-existent. He is, however, in other ways quite rational and in no way demented. Medically, he has serious illnesses and socially, there is a breakdown of his domestic and personal care.

Comment
This case has similarities with that of the Lomax couple but with certain crucial differences. In their case there was a certain medical and social

equilibrium, albeit fragile and they were prepared to accept medical and social help. Furthermore, there was no real antagonism from their neighbours or remaining relatives, merely a degree of non-interest. Mr Barlow, however, firmly refuses help. He lives in squalor that he accepts, but that results in his being rejected by both relatives and neighbours alike. The situation is one that, by normal standards, is unacceptable.

Herein lies the dilemma. Respect for Mr Barlow as a person requires that he lives his own life in his own way and is allowed to die his own death. But how far can this be taken? He is doing this within a community, particularly the community of his immediate neighbours. The stale food, the dirt, the smell and the vermin affect all who live around. How far can the sensibility and tolerance of his neighbours be offended before it is necessary to balance his freedom against theirs? Who takes these sort of decisions? There are legal provisions for dealing with this type of situation where persons are a danger to themselves or others, but these are not often implemented. The role of the doctor is often ambivalent. At what point does he/she take action? How can the relatives be included in the decision making? By this stage they have often withdrawn completely, or at least lost interest, perhaps because of old family feuds with resultant rancour. If the family doctor continues to attend, but fails to persuade Mr Barlow to take treatment, what happens if the patient dies? Is this suicide by self-neglect, or even death by medical neglect? What sort of responsibilities does the doctor have for this? An inquest would no doubt ensue.

Ethically, should the doctor tolerate the situation where an apparently rational man is slowly, of his own choice, dying, or should the doctor countermand the patient's wishes and bring in the law, with its powers of removal to a hospital or other place of safety? The situation is a reverse of the normally accepted aim of the doctor, which is to cure illness; here that opportunity is denied. In these circumstances must the GP's next duty be to others around who are affected by the patient's intransigence? What duty do doctors have to themselves to forestall allegations of allowing the patient to die, albeit slowly and naturally, because of lack of treatment? It might be that the old man is right and that treatment will make little difference; yet accepted wisdom is that treatment should be given and the doctors would normally accept this. Not to do so would possibly imperil their professional reputations. But should doctors be expected to impose their own wishes over that of their patients?

3. Mrs Jane Williamson – 'to interfere or not to interfere?'

Mrs Williamson is 89 and a widow. She lives alone in a pleasant, well-cared-for, semidetached bungalow. She has good neighbours who help her through any difficulty. Medically, she has only minor problems that she copes with herself and she is mentally alert. One morning her general practitioner is called because she has been suffering from abdominal pain through the night and feels dizzy. When the doctor examines her, her pulse is weak and rapid and her blood pressure lower than previously recorded. Abdominal examination shows her to have a swelling in the upper part of her abdomen that could be an aortic aneurysm, that is a ballooning of the main artery taking blood from the heart into the abdomen and on to the lower limbs. The doctor arranges a joint home visit with a surgeon. The surgeon confirms the general practitioner's suspicion that the patient is suffering from a leak of blood from the aneurysm and is bleeding to death. Under normal circumstances the treatment for this condition would be immediate surgery to repair the leak in the arterial wall. The surgeon, however, states that at the advanced age of 89 the operation would be extremely difficult and success would be unlikely. The operation, moreover, is a major one and even if she survived, the result would be a long period in hospital and discomfort. Mrs Williamson has no relatives apart from a sister two years older than herself who lives abroad. Her real carers and closest friends are her neighbours. The surgeon, however, leaves the decision about what to do to the general practitioner, on the grounds that it is the GP who has the best understanding of the patient.

Comment
The doctor here is faced with a very difficult decision. The patient is articulate and at this stage fully mentally alert. Under normal circumstances the first thing to do would be to discuss the situation with relatives, but it is clearly impractical to contact the older sister and probably also unwise to involve her in a burden of this kind. Moreover, how far is it right and fair to involve neighbours? The only person with whom the general practitioner can talk is, therefore, the patient herself and normally this would be the right and proper thing to do. It is, after all, her life. But looking at the situation in a humane way there is a dilemma; should the patient be told the full implications of her illness and of the options open to her, or should he say very little and allow the patient to die peacefully? Can the doctor really explain the fact that she is internally bleeding to death, that the treatment is an immediate operation that she is unlikely to survive and that even if she did so, recovery would be long and arduous? How honest could the doctor be? Is it fair to give her these options and ask her to make a decision about her own life and death?

In this case the decision is particularly pressing because the patient is becoming weaker by the hour. It is often said that general practitioners are the best people to make this sort of decision because they know their patients. Very often, however, it is almost impossible to know how a patient would react, especially at such critical moments when time is short.

Alternatively, should general practitioners make decisions about life and death on behalf of their patients? A GP is often the only one who can do so. Fortunately, in this case there is the aid of the surgeon's opinion, but can they act as a pair in this way? Removal of the disease, in this case the leaking blood vessel, could be seen to be the doctor's clear responsibility, but this is not necessarily so. Such value judgements are as important as clinical judgements. How do doctors react to them? Do they advocate risk taking? Do they leave the decisions to patients and if so, is this humane? Should they take the decisions themselves for other human beings and face the judgement of their own consciences? It may be asked what preparation doctors have for dealing with this type of dilemma and if they are at all well equipped to do so?

4. Mrs Jones – 'conflicting interests'

Grandma Jones (this is how she is known to everybody) is 65 and a widow. She is a strong matriarchal type of person who has enjoyed good health all her life and is well for her age. She is mentally alert and still continues to live life to the full. She gave up her home several years ago to live with her son and daughter-in-law in a pleasant detached house in a suburb. There are three children and with Grandma's capital they were able to move into a bigger house. There has always been some unease between Grandma Jones and her daughter-in-law. Many of the problems between the two have been associated with the younger woman's handling of her children and in particular Grandma's outspoken criticisms of it.

A crisis is precipitated in the household by the news that an unplanned fourth child is on the way. Grandma, now slightly incontinent and very embarrassed about it, is becoming an increasing burden to young Mrs Jones. Moreover, an extra room is required for the new baby, therefore pressure is placed on Grandma to move, hopefully to an old persons' home. Naturally, the elder Mrs Jones is very aggressively against this, thinking that the family house is her home and is the place where most of her capital is invested. Both women are patients of the same general practitioner and both turn to the general practitioner for help. The doctor is forced into a dilemma: to take the side of the young Mrs Jones with the problems of pregnancy and a new baby, or that of old Mrs Jones with her problems of pride and mild incontinence?

Comment

This dilemma is not uncommon for a general practitioner. Two patients, with equal rights to care, concern, advice and support have potentially conflicting interests. The issue is complicated because it is not easy to separate primarily medical aspects from social, housing and interpersonal problems. Dilemmas exist about how far the doctor's role should go. One way out would be just to treat the older person's incontinence and ignore the effects that the domestic anxieties and unpleasantness are having on her mental state and general health. Much is made in modern general practice about whole-person medicine; seeing the patient as a complete human being and taking into account environmental, social and psychological aspects.

The younger Mrs Jones confronts the general practitioner with a similar dilemma. She must also be considered as a total person. But both exist within a family and in some ways it can be argued that the doctor's responsibility is towards the whole family; after all GPs are also called *family* doctors. But does this confer the authority to act as an arbitrator? In a straightforward medical case, where there are decisions to take, the doctor's responsibilities are clear and accepted. For instance, the advice to have an inflamed appendix removed is almost always given and taken. But what about people in families? Does the doctor say 'I think, Grandma, you are the lowest priority here and that you should go' and would this be accepted? Would society see this as the doctor's role? Almost certainly not. Wise doctors, of course, would perceive these pitfalls, deal with the medical aspects and then reflect their problems back onto the family. Hopefully, by listening and facilitating discussion they would eventually enable the family to formulate their own list of solutions and come to a decision. It would then be their responsibility.

This example illustrates those aspects of medicine where decisions must be taken by those actually involved, with the doctor taking no decisive part. They lead sometimes to other ethical problems. A course of action may be agreed within a family that might, in fact, be disadvantageous to one of the members. An arrangement might be made, for example, for Grandma Jones to move into a small flat with the son financing the mortgage. This may seem to be fair, but the accommodation might be isolated, draughty, away from friends and contacts. The doctor sees the risks but is faced with a family that is obviously turning a blind eye to them. Grandma, meanwhile, is not consulted and finds herself very much worse off. Should the doctor intervene?

5. Mrs Harding – 'to condone or not to condone'

Mrs Harding is aged 75 and an ex-schoolteacher. She has always supported the idea of voluntary euthanasia and has spoken to her general practitioner about this. They have always been good friends and over the years formed a relationship of trust and respect. Sadly, Mrs Harding fell and fractured her femur whilst getting off a bus on a winter's day. She was admitted to hospital, survived an operation and made a reasonable recovery. She was discharged from the hospital, went home and the doctor was very pleased to see her progress. Within a week, however, she had the further misfortune to suffer a stroke. This resulted in Mrs

Harding being confined to bed. The opinion of the consultant was sought and it was decided that she could be nursed at home. Despite making some initial progress, Mrs Harding gradually deteriorated until she became completely bedfast. Her mental state, however, remained alert. One day she asked the doctor for a supply of sleeping tablets. Because she had not required these previously the doctor suspected that her intent was to take the entire supply in an act of voluntary euthanasia and was somewhat taken aback. Should the GP go along with this and prescribe the tablets, or refuse to co-operate and risk destroying the relationship?

Comment

There are many ethical difficulties for the doctor here. In many ways, the fact that the patient was known well was more of a hindrance than a help. In good times they had been able to communicate easily and effectively. They had talked about death and dying and made a tacit assumption about each other's position. But when the patient was faced with the reality of death and the discomfort of dying, the earlier easy communication had ceased. Neither felt able to talk about it and they resorted to subterfuge. Both, however, understood the implications. The doctor was not being asked to switch off a machine, as in the case of someone already dead, or mercifully withold treatment in the case of a moribund patient. Neither was it a case of gradually increasing the dose of a powerful narcotic in a terminal illness knowing that eventually the patient would be helped to a speedy and painless death. Mrs Harding was mentally alert, not nearing death and certainly not in pain. But life was becoming burdensome and meaningless and she wanted to die earlier than she would do if the illness ran its normal course. Although the decision, if taken, would be that of the patient and the act of swallowing the tablets would be entirely her own, and effectively be suicide, was the doctor aiding her unethically by providing the means? Would the GP be involved in the act or merely an innocent bystander? The legal situation is also difficult.

The doctor could quite legitimately say that the sedatives were prescribed in good faith and that nothing unusual was suspected. What the patient then does with the tablets is her responsibility. But had Mrs Harding swallowed the entire supply and been found dead the next morning with an empty bottle beside the bed, would the doctor feel obliged to report the matter to the coroner, so opening the possibility of a verdict of suicide? Or would a blind eye be cast on the bottle and a death certificate issued indicating a final fatal stroke? If the death is reported as suicide, has the doctor let his/her patient down? Or, perhaps, would the patient have been prepared to accept the verdict of suicide because this was her real intention?

Finally, what would be the situation if the doctor had refused to prescribe the sedatives? Although no contract had previously been made, the doctor, by refusing, was changing the terms of the relationship, saying in effect 'I do not think you are the person to take decisions about your life. I am the one who decides for you and you must trust me.' This would destroy trust and might lead Mrs Harding to seek death by other methods. But whose decision is it, if it is not the patient's? One ethical point remains. The doctor could have supplied only a small quantity of relatively harmless pills, or given the prescription to a carer with instructions about only giving the correct dosage each night. This, however, would be casuistry and does not solve the essential dilemma.

6. James Nuttall – 'risk taking'

Mr James Nuttall is aged 80 and a widower. He lives alone. His mental health is slightly failing, but he is physically in a stable condition apart from blackouts that result in occasional falls. None of these have been serious. He has had some bruises and on one occasion sustained a cut to his head that required two stitches. He is forgetful and once left his gas fire on through the night. He smokes a pipe and has had minor accidents with lighted matches. There has, however, been nothing tragic, as yet, to report. He is fundamentally contented and happy. He is seen occasionally by both his general practitioner and the health visitor. He has meals on wheels three times a week and a good caring family.

His daughter has, however, become concerned and one day consults the doctor about the state of her father. She considers that there are dangers in his handling of electricity and gas, as well as with his smoking habits and falls. All these could be potentially serious. She asserts 'It hasn't happened yet, but perhaps it will not be very long before there is an accident.' The daughter thinks that it is time that something is done. The doctor listens to all this, is sympathetic and agrees to visit Mr Nuttall with the health visitor. They find the old man in good shape. He does not know why they have come to see him because he feels well, is content in his house and sees no dangers. The doctor and health visitor examine the hazards, look at the state of the house and decide that really there is no case for advising that the old man be moved to a welfare home or sheltered housing. This is discussed with the daughter who is not satisfied and places the responsibility for her father's safety very heavily upon the doctor.

Comment

The ethical dilemma here is: what level of risk is acceptable when dealing with old persons living at home? Is it reasonable to allow the patient to live happily despite some danger? At what point do these risks become significant enough for something to be done and the patient moved to safer surroundings, even against his will? Overprotection needs to be guarded against, as well as the possibility of allowing too high a level of risk to prevail. How much should an old person's life be changed just to satisfy the overanxieties of relatives? Who are the responsible persons in this situation; the relatives and the carers, or the professional advisers? Who should take the decisions?

Can relatives be overruled? And what is the position of the doctor if something goes wrong? This is probably one of the most common ethical dilemmas to confront those working in the community and revolves round the question of who, in the last analysis, are the risk takers? Is it the patient, the relatives, or the professional advisers? This question is unanswerable and probably decides itself in practice according to the level of anxiety that each of the parties can tolerate. In any event, it is often the patient who has the least say in the eventual outcome.

7. Mrs Sarah Bagshaw – 'the dilemmas of screening'

Sarah Bagshaw is aged 75. One day she is invited to attend a screening session that aims to provide a general checkup of her health and that perhaps will detect any unmet or unreported need. She turns up cheerfully, says that she is feeling well and has no complaints to make. When the doctor examines her, however, he finds a small discharging ulcer on her breast. She says that this has been present for years and is not getting any bigger. 'I manage it myself, it is perfectly alright', she says. The doctor says that something needs to be done, and would, therefore, like to refer her to a surgeon. To the doctor it is obviously a carcinoma, albeit growing very slowly. She adamantly refuses to see a hospital specialist and, furthermore, makes the doctor promise not to tell her husband about it.

Comment

This raises the ethical issues of preventive and anticipatory care. As discussed earlier preventive care is of three types (see Chapter 10), and it is the tertiary type that mainly concerns elderly people. Screening of old people to identify established treatable illness has become fashionable. It requires intervention on the part of the doctor and is therefore in contrast to the usual patient-initiated entry into medical care. This means that extra responsibilities are placed on the doctor. The screening must be reliable in identifying the conditions it sets out to discover. It must be possible to do something positive when these conditions are found. With elderly patients, the method of screening is variable, but usually involves taking a history, carrying out a full physical examination and undertaking certain tests on the blood and urine. This is a reasonably reliable method of diagnosing unreported but established medical conditions.

Screening, however, raises ethical problems. If something incurable is discovered, how far does the doctor carry investigation and treatment, especially if the patient was previously unaware of the problem? Obviously, treatable conditions such as diabetes mellitus and heart failure need attention. But what of Mrs Bagshaw, the patient with cancer of the breast? Should the doctor comply with her request to do nothing and, furthermore, not discuss the situation with her husband or relatives? Should the doctor communicate with all these people secretly and break the contract of confidentiality that the patient has presumed? Is it lacking in care not to give the patient the benefit of referral and the prospect of treatment? The question, to some extent, rests on the mandate that the patient gave the doctor when permission was given to carry out a screening procedure. But the patient does not always understand the full implications of this mandate. Does it imply acceptance of treatment and advice, or is this a different mandate that needs renegotiation? Clearly in Mrs Bagshaw's case, renegotiation was needed in the light of circumstances. The doctor who conducts the screen must recognize that this is a possibility and respect the patient's wishes. It, nevertheless, can result in dilemmas to which there are no straightforward solutions.

8. Mr and Mrs Fletcher – 'captive spouse'

Mr and Mrs Fletcher live in a terraced house in an area that has 'seen better days'. She is aged 69 and he is 72. Mrs Fletcher has suffered from multiple sclerosis for the past 20 years, is now bedfast and becoming increasingly dependent. As time has passed she has developed heart failure and increased forgetfulness. Mr Fletcher is doing all the housework and shopping as well as nursing his wife. His health is holding, but only just. His social life is non-existent and he has become totally captive to his house and task.

Mrs Fletcher develops pneumonia. The doctor advises that she be admitted to hospital but her husband refuses, insists that he can cope and, moreover, provide better nursing. His wife supports him in this decision. The doctor is reluctant to agree because he perceives that Mr Fletcher's health is beginning to fail and that it would be risky to expose him to the extra strain. However, Mr and Mrs Fletcher's wishes are respected and full nursing services are arranged. Initially, the patient responds to treatment, but after three weeks of arduous and painstaking care by her husband, she relapses. Hospital admission is still rejected by Mr Fletcher. The doctor now seriously asks himself whether or not he should continue to treat Mrs Fletcher's bronchopneumonia or allow events to take their natural course.

Comment

This is a real dilemma. Withholding antibiotics would probably allow her a peaceful death in her own home nursed by her husband. For his part, Mr Fletcher would feel that he had done his duty and cared for his wife to the best of his ability. The doctor might feel that of the two lives, the most valuable one to save is that of Mr Fletcher. Mrs Fletcher could be admitted to hospital, but totally against the wishes of both. Obviously a high level of help in the house can be arranged, but what about the antibiotics? The usual action taken by a doctor would be to prescribe, with the intention of coping with the husband as and when necessary. How much, however, is the decision the doctor's and how far should he/she discuss the possible courses of action with both the patient and her husband? Mr Fletcher undoubtedly realizes the consequences for his own health of nursing his wife in this way. Is he implying that he too wants to die? The doctor may sense this and find him/herself colluding in a situation of considerable human significance.

9. Mr John Fairweather – 'help or no help'

John Fairweather, a widower, is aged 80 and lives in sheltered accommodation. He enjoys the company of other residents and is visited occasionally by relatives. He suffered from a stroke several years ago and is left with a partial paralysis of his right side. Despite this he walks reasonably well with a Zimmer frame, although he does not go out.

Mr Fairweather also has severe osteoarthritis of his left hip, which compounds his mobility problems and causes him a considerable amount of pain. His doctor treats this symptomatically with pain-relieving tablets. The patient, however, desperately wants to have a hip replacement, which he considers would relieve his pain and improve his mobility. His doctor and the orthopaedic surgeon to whom he is referred were against this on the grounds of the previous stroke and the dangers of an anaesthetic. These problems are discussed fully with both the patient and his relatives. However, because of Mr Fairweather's persistence, the operation is eventually performed. He is discharged from hospital six weeks later, is bedfast, with pressure sores and urinary incontinence. His doctor is horrified.

Comment

There are two problems here. At what point should the doctor intervene when a patient is subjected, or in this case subjects himself, to procedures or treatment that carry the risk of causing further harm to his health? Can the doctor say 'no' when the risk is obviously considerable, or is the patient to be allowed to proceed? In this case the risks of the operation were clear and it was obviously an extreme step to take if the aim was only pain relief. The surgeon needed to balance the risks with the possible benefits. In this case, pressure from the patient and relatives probably influenced the decision and the risk was taken. Was it ethical for the general practitioner to refer the patient in the first place when there were severe doubts about the advisability of surgery?

The second problem is the doctor's reaction to the patient's condition on return from hospital. Were the bedsores a result of poor and careless nursing? Should the GP make a fuss, or quietly work to improve the patient's condition now that he has returned home? At all events the doctor might well ask the question 'How much real help have I been to this old patient?'

DISCUSSION

Six ethical dilemmas are illustrated by these case histories. They concern: responsibility, priorities, information, confidentiality, collusion and intervention. They will be dealt with separately though there is inevitable interlinkage. Few situations in medicine are as simple as first appears and often several ethical problems impinge on each other.

Responsibility

The problem with responsibility is: where does it finally rest? As has been seen, it is possible for an old couple (Case 1) to be living in conditions that an outsider would describe as intolerable and yet are perfectly acceptable to them. It can be argued that the responsibility as to how an old person lives rests with that person, but once the doctor enters the situation it could also be argued that he/she, by accepting it, may also share some of the responsibility. (The doctor is also colluding in these circumstances, but this will be considered later.) Similarly, relatives sometimes complain about the risks taken by an old man living alone (Case 6). Who should accept responsibility for these risks? The relatives want the professional carers to do so, whereas the latter put the onus on the relatives. The patient's feelings may not even be considered.

The risks to professional workers who exercise these responsibilities are obvious and much fudging of the issues often takes place. In the final analysis the actions of reasonable people having the skills normally possessed by members of their profession are seen as the norm. If too much weight is placed on autonomy, the patient may be exposed to unacceptable risks. By accepting the patient's view, is the doctor acting unreasonably in allowing potential hazards to develop?

Thus ethical issues can impinge on legal issues and the resultant dilemmas are hard to resolve.

Priorities

The next dilemma concerns priorities. They can concern balancing the priorities of one patient against those of another, or of a patient against those of relatives, neighbours and society itself. The conflicting needs of the old lady and her daughter-in-law (Case 4) were very starkly presented to the family doctor. How far should the doctor interfere when decisions, taken quite justifiably by the family, are ethically unfair or medically detrimental to one of the parties? Again, the patient who chooses to live in neglect and refuse treatment (Case 2) has theoretically every right to do so. But what are the rights of the neighbours? Should the doctor bring in the law and have the patient removed to a place of care, or turn a blind eye and leave the neighbours, who are perhaps not the doctor's concern, to make complaints and demand action for themselves?

Furthermore, at what point do doctors need to consider their own positions? Do they need to safeguard their reputations in the neighbourhood and secure themselves against possible action in the courts (thereby relieving themselves of the burden of unacceptable anxiety)? Fortunately these situations are rare and the task of solving them can be shared with others who do not have the same clinical responsibilities. Nevertheless, in borderline cases the dilemma can be real.

Information

The question of information is usually concerned with how much should be told. The dilemma of Mrs Williamson was of this type (Case 3).

What is the ethical position of the doctor when informing patients that they are about to die? Stark situations like the one described are probably rare, but when an urgent decision needs taking that involves assessment of risk, what factors influence the degree of involvement of the patient? Communication is the keystone of medical practice and involves giving information, but how far should this be withheld to preserve other important matters such as a patient's dignity and peace of mind? Is it right for a doctor to take crucial decisions on a patient's behalf without fully informing the patient about all the facts, even if these are very distressing? The question often poses itself as whether to interfere or not, the wisest course often being the latter. In practice the patient, and if present the relatives, often want the doctor to take the decisions anyway. They place themselves in a physician's hands to relieve themselves of decision, responsibility and perhaps possible future guilt.

Confidentiality

How far confidentiality should be taken is a major issue and involves all age groups. A poignant case was that of the patient who wanted to take her own life, as an act of voluntary euthansia, when life had become intolerable to her (Case 5). If the doctor had colluded, how ethical would this have been? And how far should the doctor have gone in respecting her confidentiality? Making a false declaration on a death certificate is unlawful, but could there be instances in which the doctor might consider it a duty to the deceased patient to make one?

The lady who had breast cancer and wanted nobody to know about it also presented an example of the dilemma of confidentiality (Case 7). Would it be ethically wrong for the doctor to inform her husband against her consent, when there were overwhelming reasons for doing it? At what point is confidentiality broken and information passed? When is it ethical to break a confidence? These are unresolved questions. Guidelines may be available, but in the end the doctor is often alone when taking such decisions.

Collusion

The problems of collusion have already been touched on. The most obvious example is colluding with a patient who wishes to accept the unacceptable, as in the case of Mr Barlow (Case 2). But collusion is also possible in relation to information. Relatives often ask a doctor not to tell a patient about the true nature of an illness. What if the patient wants to know and asks outright? Should the doctor respect the collusion sought by the relatives or is it ethically a duty to inform the patient? Very occasionally collusion between professional colleagues may occur. In the case of John Fairweather, where there may have been poor care following the operation, resulting in bedsores, should the doctor make this an issue or simply be concerned with the immediate tasks? Is the latter course unethical collusion? Where does a general practitioner's loyalty lie in these circumstances? Again, the ethical judgement remains very much with the personal conscience of the doctor. A subtle situation also occurs when the doctor 'colludes' with him/herself. How often are issues avoided and actions taken that are not absolutely in the patient's best interests? Maybe the doctor's own interests of convenience, comfort or reduction in worry can result in temptation. A patient who is obviously going to prove difficult to manage can be admitted to hospital, although home care is theoretically possible and perhaps best for the patient.

Intervention

With the ever-increasing numbers of elderly patients, general practice will concern itself more and more with the care of patients suffering from chronic illness. A dilemma that will arise is how active should practitioners be in treatment and intervention? Sometimes the effect of active treatment may be more harmful than the problem itself. Many patients are admitted to hospital with iatrogenic diseases, conditions that have been brought on by the effects of treatment. An example is John Fair-weather and his hip operation (Case 9). Should the patient alone decide these issues, having heard about the risks and possible outcomes? It is sometimes difficult for the doctor to be sure, despite much discussion with the patient and relatives, that a clear understanding of all the relevant issues has been achieved. How ethical is it for doctors to proceed against their own judgement? There are situations in which, obviously, they should argue strongly against certain actions. But there are also grey areas where risks are hard to evaluate and outcomes are unpredictable.

Anticipatory care is now in vogue: searching out previously untreated or unreported illness so that it can be alleviated. The ethical issues here also need clarification. Having found an untreated illness, what then? As a case described earlier highlights, patients may not want treatment (Case 7). Is it a situation to be accepted and no help given? Ethically, should doctors accept this even though they are colluding with the patient, perhaps against what the doctor perceives as his/her better interests?

Modern general practice is aware of these ethical dilemmas and accepts the need to take them into consideration when taking decisions. Consultations often give rise to ethical dilemmas, but, happily, most are resolved without too much difficulty. In the final analysis most of these issues are decided on considerations based on respect for the patient. It is only when the doctor is presented with *conflicting* needs that real difficulties arise.

This chapter is based on one written by the author in *Medical Ethics and Elderly People* (Elford, 1987). In that work a response to the ethical issues posed in this chapter is given by Dr W. Donald Hudson, formerly Reader in Moral Philosophy, University of Exeter.

REFERENCE

R.J. Elford (ed.) (1987) *Medical Ethics and Elderly People*, Churchill Livingstone, London.

21 *The dying patient*

Death is the logical end to old age and the care of the dying old person is the final service provided by the doctor throughout the ageing process. Many other people are necessarily involved, but at this stage the role of the doctor is usually crucial. Often the relationship that has been built up over the years has turned to friendship and nursing an old person who has come to the end of a long and interesting life should be a fulfilling experience. Sadly, it is becoming less common for old people to die in their own homes and these days most people die in hospital or in a hospice. But even when this happens, a large part of the terminal illness involves being at home where the patient continues to be under the care of the family doctor.

Most people fear death or at least the act of dying, but many elderly people regard it with philosophical resignation rather than anger and frustration. 'I've had enough, doctor and I'm ready to go' has been said many times by the very old and death is often a quick and happy event.

However, with a younger patient real emotional and spiritual problems and dilemmas sometimes confront the doctor. Previous knowledge of the personality of the patient may help to understand some of these and the doctor should certainly always be prepared to discuss fears and anxieties. Family doctors are often in a special position to recognize these because of the patient's previous emotional reaction to illness. Even though dying, the patient still remains a living individual human being, and deserves to be treated as such. The real test of a relationship comes when the decision has to be taken as to whether or not to tell the patient that the illness is in fact terminal. The decision rests on circumstances. Sometimes it is unnecessary to say anything, and this is true particularly of elderly people, because they are often aware that life is slipping away. They know and accept that death is inevitable and this should be respected. There is a silent understanding between patient and doctor and both realize what is happening.

In other cases, particularly involving younger people, it may be apparent that the patient is reluctant to face the reality and does not want to know the truth. In these situations the doctor should tactfully avoid telling the full facts, but at the same time be careful not to destroy trust by making statements that lack credibility. Much can be done by discussing the causation of the symptoms and making sure that these are effectively relieved. This course is possibly the most frequent one taken and it may be that it is unnecessary and cruel to spell out in precise terms to the patient that death is approaching. The doctor should find out relatives' wishes and if they want silence this should be acknowledged. However, if someone really wants and needs to know the full nature of their illness and its likely course, particularly if their mental and emotional state is balanced, I personally think the truth should be told. A person often needs this knowledge to make certain adjustments and to prepare for the inevitable. The dying person may need to re-establish certain relationships, to come to terms with his or her past life and to be happy with the arrangements made for family and friends.

Judging *when* to tell may be difficult. Dying people may go through distinct emotional changes. They may at first show strong disbelief that anything of serious consequence is happening and it is at this stage that pressures are brought to bear on the doctor for second opinions and hospital admission. This is a stage of denial. There follows a stage of anger and this is sometimes directed against the doctor, who is held to be responsible in some way for the illness and its incurable nature. Linked with this are the emotions of depression and fear as patients realize that life is coming to an end. Gradually, however, there is acceptance of the situation and a more serene mood takes over. It is at this stage that patients are perhaps ready for the whole truth and prepared to come to terms with unresolved problems. This is an important stage at which old people, in particular, arrive more quickly and they do not necessarily pass through the earlier stages described. Hopefully, eventually, serenity is achieved and it can be an impressive and beautiful human experience.

The doctor has four main tasks when confronted with a dying patient: first to establish the diagnosis, second, to alleviate distress, third, to support the family and finally, to co-ordinate other services. These apply of course to all ages and not just to the very old. The stages will be described separately.

DIAGNOSIS

It is necessary to be absolutely certain that the diagnosis is correct and that death is inevitable. A doctor must not only be satisfied as to the incurable and fatal nature of the illness, usually cancer, but must also satisfy the relatives. If there is any doubt, a second opinion should be taken but if possible, subjection of a weary old person to intensive investigations should be avoided. Once everyone has faith in the correctness of the diagnosis and the eventual outcome, it is surprising how much easier management becomes. Nothing is more difficult than a family who will not accept the inevitable.

ALLEVIATION OF DISTRESS

The doctor has a wide range of 'weapons' for relieving distress and is aided in this by the nurse in the team. The presence of the doctor and nurse is a very important therapeutic factor, providing support and comfort to a dying patient. The doctor must provide continuing care, calling to see the patient regularly; towards the end, this visiting must be every day or even several times in one day. The visiting must be reliable and relatives should not need to call or send for the doctor. Communication with the patient is very important; there may be no need to talk always about deep matters but the opportunity should be there to discuss and listen. Alleviation of distress usually means palliative treatment of symptoms and adequate relief of pain. Mental problems also need attention. In younger patients, depression and frustration may predominate, but this is not common with the very old and confusion may be the prevailing symptom.

Relief of pain

Pain is the symptom that is most feared by most patients. Perhaps it is not such a dominant symptom as might be imagined in a dying old person and it is probable that about 60% of cancer patients die without significant pain. Where it is present, however, it demands effective relief. It is important to define the type and site of the pain because this might affect the analgesic given. Good treatment should anticipate pain because if it returns before the next dose of analgesic, it becomes harder to control. If, however, appropriate analgesics are given regularly then pain can be completely controlled in most cases, and the dose of analgesics can be kept low. Once the pain is properly controlled the patient no longer has to ask for relief. The aim should be to provide a full night's sleep without pain, to control pain at rest and to control pain on movement. The first two are always possible, the last one not always so. It is essential to beware of giving drugs only on demand. This means that analgesics are only given when the patient is already complaining of pain. The first essential is that instructions must be clear and the analgesics given at specified intervals so that once pain is controlled it does not return. The initial stage of pain control is with simple drugs that are familiar: aspirin, paracetamol with dextropropoxyphene or paracetamol alone. If these fail, there should be no hesitation in immediately going on to something stronger, for instance, dihydrocodeine tartrate (DF118) 30 mg. If the pain is severe, it is necessary to turn to the opiate group of drugs. Morphine and diamorphine are undoubtedly the most effective. Phenazocine (Narphen) and dipipanone (Diconal) are sometimes used as alternatives, the former if constipation is a problem.

It is important that the rationale for using the opiate group of drugs is completely understood. It is wrong to think that morphine is an addictive hallucinogenic drug needing to be given in larger and larger dosage because of tolerance. It is usual to start with an oral preparation every four hours because this is how long the effect lasts. The dose needs adjusting until effective relief of pain is achieved. The dosage can then be continued for as long as two years with no need for any alterations. In certain cases dependency arises after several weeks of administration, but this does not usually cause any difficulties. When pain relief has been satisfactorily achieved, a change to long-acting preparations is helpful on an eight-hourly basis. Where vomiting is a problem or the patient cannot swallow the tablet or liquid, injection, usually of diamorphine, is indicated, and the dose modified accordingly. An alternative is morphine suppositories, but these are not reliable and again, the dose needs to be carefully reviewed. Syringe drivers are also used at home for opiate injections and obviates the need for four-hourly injections. Their use, however, does demand experience.

There are two important side effects of opiates: nausea and constipation. The choice of antiemetic is important and prochlorperazine (Stemetil) or perphenazine (Fentazin) are preferable. It should be remembered that the dosage of these drugs should not necessarily be increased along with the increased dose of opiate, because then the patient may suffer from extrapyramidal side effects of too much antiemetic. Constipation always occurs with long-term opiate treatment and needs careful control. Any one of these drugs will need a simple laxative from the second day and suppositories are often helpful in this respect.

Two drugs often used in the past for pain relief have dropped out of fashion. These are pentazocine and pethidine. The latter has too short a half-life and frequently causes vomiting. The old-fashioned Brompton's mixture is now not often used. Cocaine does not have any analgesic effect and was often responsible for the hallucinogenic and addictive effects of the mixture. Less severe pain can be controlled by buprenorphine (Temgesic), which has recently become very popular because of the ease of administration. It has one drawback, however, in that in quite a lot of patients it causes vomiting.

Particular kinds of pain need special kinds of technique. Bone pain is helped by non-steroidal anti-inflammatory drugs, for instance aspirin or flurbiprofen. These can be augmented by radiation or quinine nerve block. Soft-tissue pain and nerve compression can be helped by morphine together with prednisolone. Pain arising from raised intercranial pressure can again be helped by morphine, combined with dexamethasone. Pain produced by oedema can be helped by a diuretic and, sometimes, a steroid. Antibiotics are necessary when infection is contributing to the pain. Where muscle spasm is present a muscle relaxant such as diazepam can often prove helpful.

Relief of other symptoms

A dying patient may suffer from a wide range of symptoms and complications. Common problems are cough, vomiting, breathlessness and
constipation. A full description of the routine management of these
problems is not given here. An excellent review however is given in
Derek Doyle's book *Domiciliary Terminal Care* (1987) and should be read by
all those providing care to dying patients (see references, p. 266).

General instructions to patients

It is necessary to tell patients and their carers that regular administration
of pain-relieving drugs is important. Sometimes it is helpful to put these
instructions in writing. Both the patient and relatives should be informed
about possible side-effects, explaining that these are usually only temporary, but that the doctor needs informing so that if appropriate, a
change in drug can be made. It is especially important in this connection
to mention drowsiness and confusion so that the doctor knows when this
is happening.

SUPPORT TO FAMILIES

Apart from the patient, the doctor is faced with caring for the relatives.
Even with a very elderly person it is sometimes hard to accept that death
is inevitable. The doctor must again reassure them that the diagnosis is
correct and that no cure is available. Even so, disbelief is sometimes slow
to be resolved but acceptance of the situation is eventually achieved and
much love then goes into the continuing care and attention given to the
patient. Relatives need not only emotional support but also practical help
with the management of domestic affairs. Although about to die, the
patient still needs a full range of services. The doctor is probably the
only person in a position to arrange and co-ordinate these.

CO-ORDINATION OF OTHER SERVICES

The *nursing care* for the dying patient is provided by the community
nursing service. The general principles of home nursing are described
elsewhere and apply with particular regard to such problems as pressure
sores and incontinence. Supervision of treatment and pain relief are also
very much the nurse's task. Special problems such as disposal of soiled
dressings may occur. They should be burned if possible, but otherwise
they can be wrapped in a polythene bag and placed in a dustbin. Special
arrangements can be made with local authority cleansing departments for
this type of disposal. Offensive smells and odours are also sometimes

a problem but fortunately, modern deodorants and air fresheners can overcome this. Quite often a 24-hour nursing service is necessary and district health authorities may be able to provide this. When patients are dying from malignant disease, the Marie Curie Memorial Foundation Day and Night Nursing Service is available for this purpose. The nurse is very much involved in general support and encouragement to the family. By the very nature of the problem, a strong bond of trust builds up between herself and the patient. The family may also become very dependent on the nurse and she should accept this in the knowledge that it is self-limiting. Once the patient has died, the nurse should attend to the body and dispose of soiled linen. Any unused drugs should be destroyed and equipment removed.

In this country *social workers* have not been much involved in dealing with the problems of patients dying at home. Any pressing social problem has usually been dealt with by the doctor or nurse. These days, with economic, social and family problems increasing, and the added number of old people living alone without adequate support, the social worker is increasingly likely to be involved. Practical assistance such as home help, laundry service, special aids and adaptations can be necessary. The difficulties involved, however, in managing this type of situation where there is no family help do often make it impossible for such patients to die at home and hospital admission becomes necessary. This reduces the opportunity for social-worker involvement. It may be necessary to provide social support for a family that needs to deal with such problems as finance, the care of children and the disposal of effects. Counselling of a particularly upset member of the family may well be an important contribution made by the social worker, although the doctor must also be very much involved in helping with this type of situation.

Much help can also be had from voluntary organizations in sustaining a family nursing a dying relative. Social workers are usually able to locate these sources of help. BACUP is a patient-information service that aims to help people by giving practical advice and support. Neighbours and friends are often invaluable in giving relatives a break and undertaking such tasks as shopping. Ministers and priests should also be brought in at an early stage and can bring practical and spiritual help to the family.

The hospice movement

The hospice movement started with the opening, in 1967, of St Christopher's Hospice in London. The founder, Dame Cicely Saunders, there carried out her pioneering work on the care of terminally ill patients. About 150 hospice-type units now exist. Some are National Health Service specialist units but many are charitable foundations. Most hospices have in-patient care, which aims to provide symptom control and family relief for those terminally ill. These is also sometimes opportunity for active rehabilitation. Medical advice may also be available about patients who are being nursed at home. Continuing care at home is also provided by a system of home-support nurses known as MacMillan nurses. This service is funded by the National Society for Cancer Relief. The Mac-Millan Nursing Service is involved in liaison between the primary-care team and the hospice unit and is able to offer specialist nursing advice. Emotional support and counselling for carers and patients is also available. It is often helpful to refer the patients to this service at an early stage so that planned palliative care can be achieved. The hospice movement is not, therefore, only concerned with admitting dying patients but is also very much concerned with keeping people out of hospital and in the community, especially when pain has been controlled. Several admissions may be necessary and an introduction into the hospice at an early stage is often an advantage. The hospice can also lend useful pieces of apparatus that would not otherwise be available.

SELF-UNDERSTANDING

Everyone who has to care for dying patients must also come to terms with their own attitude to death. It is an event clouded with mystery and easily relegated to the background of consciousness. For the religious it marks a beginning, but for the unbeliever the unknown. How should doctors, nurses and social workers react to a patient's spiritual need? If they are religious themselves and know the patient's attitudes, perhaps they can be involved in giving spiritual comfort, but for most this is a difficult task. It is probably best to leave these matters to the professional clergy. Patients do get comfort from religion at this stage and turn to it sometimes for the first time in their lives. An understanding and kindly member of the clergy can bring great benefit in this type of situation.

Sometimes, however, patients want to talk about these matters with a doctor or nurse and this can bring a professional carer face to face with the realities of personal attitudes and feelings towards death. It is sometimes helpful to remember the works of John Donne, the famous Dean of St Paul's, who wrote the following immortal words:

Now this bell tolling softly for another says to me,
Thou must die.
No man is an island entire of itself,
Every man is a piece of the continent a part of the main,
If a clod be washed by the sea, Europe is the less.
Any man's death diminishes me because I am involved in Mankind,
And therefore never seek to know for whom the bell tolls,
It tolls for thee.

REFERENCE

Doyle, D. (1987) *Domiciliary Terminal Care. A Handbook for Doctors and Nurses,* Churchill Livingstone, Edinburgh.

USEFUL READING

Kubler-Ross, E. (1969) *On Death and Dying,* Tavistock, London.
Lammerton, R. (1973) *Care of the Dying,* Priory Press, Hove.
Murray Parkes, C. (1972) *Bereavement,* Tavistock, London.
Raven, R.W. (1975) *The Dying Patient,* Pitman Medical, London.
Saunders, S. (ed.) (1978) *Management of Terminal Illness,* Edward Arnold, London.

22   *Conclusions*

The concluding chapter of the first edition of this book (written ten years ago) examined future developments and possible problems in caring for elderly persons. Clinics for elderly people based on general practice were forecast, and also the increasing burdens that would be placed on family and carers. Further research was envisaged especially on the economic implications of the expected increase in the numbers of elderly people. It was thought that changes in attitudes were necessary amongst professional carers towards elderly people, with appropriate educational input to achieve this. One sentence revealingly hinted that elderly people themselves would accept responsibilities for self-care and suggested that they should integrate and not segregate.

Looking back at the last ten years there have been some developments in these areas. Special clinics, although not a widespread feature of general practice, do exist and the idea of a practice having one is no longer outrageous. The problems of carers are much more fully appreciated. Little research, however, has been undertaken into the delivery of care for elderly people and the economic implications are still far from being understood. There are some changes in attitudes, but negativism is still a significant block to the development of better systems of care, and much still needs to be done educationally. Old people themselves probably now have a more positive approach to ageing, and the news is good about overall health status.

There have, however, been significant changes that were not foreseen. New ideas have emerged about preventive care. Comprehensive screening has, on the whole, given way to selective screening and opportunistic screening. Anticipatory care, with its emphasis on health promotion as well as disease prevention is now important and accepted. The need for interface care when patients move from one system to another is clearly identified. The ethical issues associated with community care are also now much better understood. The introduction of the Diploma in Geriatric Medicine examination is a stimulus to extending educational facilities amongst doctors. A major development has been the privatization of nursing homes and rest homes, thus changing dramatically the provision of long-stay care. This has revolutionized the hospital-bed situation, but has also brought problems. How long it will last is a debatable point.

Looking into the future, education is likely to become vitally significant. Health care of elderly people is now established as a discipline, with academic departments in most United Kingdom medical schools. All undergraduates have geriatric medicine in their curriculum. The exposure of students to care of elderly people in the community is also developing, through academic departments of general practice or primary care. The mandatory three-year postgraduate vocational-training requirement before achieving principal status is producing much better equipped general practitioners. Most trainees get geriatric medicine hospital experience at senior house officer level, and this is to be encouraged. The one-year experience as a trainee in general practice has allowed the young doctor to learn about the care of old people at home. Hopefully, day-release courses supplement this learning. Continuing postgraduate education in general practice is not as well developed and there is an urgent need for this in the United Kingdom. Other disciplines, including nursing, social work and the therapies also need educational input into their training about health care of elderly people and this is developing. In all areas, attitudinal as well as technical awareness need to be stimulated.

As this book is published, a nodal point has probably been reached in the evolution of primary care in the UK, and this will have important implications for elderly people. The White Paper on Primary Care, the Cumberlege Report, the Griffiths Report on Community Care and others all signal major changes. The wide examination of the health services currently being undertaken by Government may indicate even more fundamental changes. The White Paper supports preventive activity in primary care and this may well be helpful in the case of elderly people, but other changes, such as increasing competition between doctors, may be harmful. Neighbourhood nursing schemes may well remove from old people the benefit of a known practice-attached district nurse. The wide remit given by the Griffiths Report to local authorities for the provision of long-term care of elderly people is very dependent upon financial resources and experienced management. The place of private capital in this needs to be clarified.

The indications are that there will be a shift of care for old people from the hospital- (secondary-) care system to the community. The dangers are that this will take place inappropriately and inadequately. Much is now understood about looking after old people, including the nature of their needs, especially those who are very old. Indeed it is with the very old that we should be presently concerned. The relative increase of the old old in the population over the next decade will mean an increased demand for services. Unfortunately, the organizational structure available in the community is not ideal for undertaking this task. The tripartite management system, health authority, local authority and Family Practitioner Committee, is inappropriate for providing the integrated care system that is essential when caring for old people. Sensible planning, proper communication, effective allocation of resources and efficient use of available staff all demand a unified system of management. None of the reports and papers have addressed this question. The final sentence of the 1979 edition of this book stated: 'In the community the full resources of the medical and social team must be integrated and so organised that the lessons learned over the past few years are fully utilised to improve the standards of care given to our old people.' Will it be different in the next ten years?

Appendix

Anticipatory care checklist suitable for a Lloyd George envelope

Date:	Assessment by:

Name:	Age:
Address:	DOB:
	MSD:

Telephone:

Next of kin	Carer
Tel:	Tel:

Physical/Mental			Other
General condition Good Fair Poor	*Hearing*	Normal/needs hearing aid	
	Eyesight	Normal/needs glasses	Weight
Mental state Normal Early dementia	*Continence:*	Urine Bowels	BP
Depressed Confused	*Heart/lung:*	Breathless Chest pain	Urine
			Hb
Mobility Normal Restricted	*Skin:*	Ulcer rash	Blood sugar
Needs help	*Teeth:*	Dentures Own teeth	
	Feet:		ESR

Major problems	*Drugs*	*Social service*
		Vol. organization

Social state	ADL	*Next assessment*
Safety	Shopping	
Alone	Housework	*Action*
Housefast	Hobbies	
Heating	Bathing	
Support	Cooking	
House type		
Comment	*Comment*	

Hospital

Action taken	Date: Follow up	Date: Follow up	Date: Follow up
Nothing Doctor District nurse Health visitor Social worker Home help Chiropodist Referral Age Concern Other			

Date	Notes

Index

and special utensils 145
Obesity 145, 230
Obsessive neurosis 226–27
Occlusion 210
Occupation 117
Occupational therapists 77, 79, 126, 154, 193, 201, 202
Oceania 10
Oedema 46, 121, 187
Oesophageal mobility 141
Office of Population Censuses and Surveys (OPCS) 8, 10
Old peoples' homes, *see* 'Part III' homes
Opiate drugs 256–57
    side effects 257
Opit, L.J. 68, 187
Opportunistic case-finding 128–30
Opportunistic intervention 151
Opsite 204
Optical services 126
Opticians 72, 83, 96
Orme M. 212
Orthopaedics 161
Osscular adhesions 236
Ossicles 236
Osteoarthritis 51, 53, 119, 229, 249
Osteomalacia 141, 229
Osteopathy 188
Osteoporosis 45, 51, 229
Otosclerosis 236
Out-patient departments 87, 161
Out-patient referral 125
Over-eighties pension 37
Owner occupation 24, 33

Paget's disease 229, 237
Papilloedema 212
Papillomata 49
Paracetamol 256
Paramedical staff 133
Paraphrenia 225
Parkinsonism 147, 230
Parkinson's Disease Society 84
'Part III' homes 2, 28–29, 67, 84, 94–96, 99, 184
    admission to 94, 95
    assessment before admission 94–95
Pathy, M.S.J. 48
Patient participation 196–97
Patient record systems 98

Pattie, A.H. 155
Pension premium 37
Pensions 23, 26, 30–33, 36–37, 57
    Additional 36–37
    Basic 36
    Graduated 37
    Industrial Injuries Disablement 41
    Invalidity 39
    Over-eighties 30
    State Earnings Related Pension Scheme (SERPS) 36–37
    War dependents' 41
    War widows' 41
    Widows' 40
Pentazocine 257
Perforated ear-drum 236
Perkins, E.R. 17, 112
Perphenazine 257
Personality changes 226–27
Pethidine 257
Pets 25–26
Pharmaceutical services 72
Pharmacists 73, 74, 184, 194
Phenazocine 256
Phenformin 217
Phenothiazone tranquillizers 147
Phenylbutazone 142
Phenytoin 142
Physical handicap 59
Physically handicapped children 59
Physiotherapy 74, 75, 79, 80, 87, 126, 154, 187, 193, 201, 209, 231
Pipe smoking 26
Platelet function 211
Pneumococcal vaccines 136
Pneumonia 78, 136, 248
Police 74
Political purges 8
Polymyalgia rheumatica 191, 229–30
Polypharmacy 187
Poor Law 90, 96
Population projections 10–12
Postal questionnaires 131–33, 134
Postgraduate education 263
Postural hypotension 232
Poverty 57, 130
Power of attorney 227
Practice managers 74
Practice nurses 74, 128, 129, 195, 202
Practice registers 181
Practice staff 74
Practice strategy 195–97